Thales Coelho de Alvarenga

Search for porcine parvovirus and Mycoplasma hyopneumonie in pigs

Thales Coelho de Alvarenga

Search for porcine parvovirus and Mycoplasma hyopneumonie in pigs

SEARCH FOR SWINE PARVOVIRUS AND Mycoplasma hyopneumoniae IN PIGS WITH SWINE CIRCOVIROSIS FROM THE STATE OF GOIÁS

Imprint

Any brand names and product names mentioned in this book are subject to trademark, brand or patent protection and are trademarks or registered trademarks of their respective holders. The use of brand names, product names, common names, trade names, product descriptions etc. even without a particular marking in this work is in no way to be construed to mean that such names may be regarded as unrestricted in respect of trademark and brand protection legislation and could thus be used by anyone.

Cover image: www.ingimage.com

This book is a translation from the original published under ISBN 978-613-9-63165-0.

Publisher:
Sciencia Scripts
is a trademark of
Dodo Books Indian Ocean Ltd. and OmniScriptum S.R.L publishing group

120 High Road, East Finchley, London, N2 9ED, United Kingdom
Str. Armeneasca 28/1, office 1, Chisinau MD-2012, Republic of Moldova, Europe
Printed at: see last page
ISBN: 978-620-7-76989-6

SUMMARY

ACKNOWLEDGMENTS

My sincere thanks go to my family, especially my mother, Maria Célia Alvarenga, for all the years she has been by my side, and for her constant encouragement and support in the arduous struggle to achieve my life's projects. To my sister, Tatiany Coelho Alvarenga, and my nephew, Pedro Fernandes Gatti, for awakening in me the taste of unconditional love.

To my advisor, Wilia Marta Elsner Diederichsen de Brito, who, in addition to her brilliant guidance, proved to be a helping hand at many times, and was even my confidante in a particularly stormy circumstance in my personal life. I would like to thank her for her affection, understanding, availability and also for the "calls", which I am aware were made with the sole intention of making me grow.

To Patricia Soares and Tatyane Penha Sales, without whom I wouldn't have had so much information about the animals studied here.

To my dear biochemistry teacher, Maria de Lourdes Breseghelo, who, during my undergraduate studies, was a true mother of spirit in my academic life, having been one of the first people to believe in my intellectual potential, awakening in me the will to win.

The School of Veterinary Science and Zootechnics (EVZ) at UFG, for all the knowledge offered to me, and to the valuable professors Cintia Silva Minafra e Resende, Iolanda Aparecida Nunes, José Henrique Stringhini, Maria Auxiliadora Andrade and Marcos Barcellos Café, whose students I had the opportunity to teach at this institution. In particular, my eternal gratitude goes to the noble professor Valéria de Sá Jayme, a substantial source of wisdom and inspiration in times of learning, and a supportive base for encouraging the art of living, I lack words to describe my admiration and gratitude to her, thank you for being part of my story.

To my friends Lindomar Marques de Oliveira and Ênio Eduardo Basilio for putting up with me and encouraging me, to my seminar friend Micaela Guidotti Takeuchi and especially to Ricardo Luiz Clemente.

To the collaborators at the Biological Institute of São Paulo, Vera Lettice de Azevedo Ruiz, Alessandra Figueiredo de Castro Nassar, Josete Garcia Bersano and Renato Akio Ogata, who contributed greatly to the completion of this dissertation.

To Andréia Oliveria de Santana, administrative servant in the postgraduate sector of the EVZ at UFG, for her patience, promptness and attention in dealing with my requests.

To my dogs, Suzy, Branca, Brenda and Bruce for their companionship and moments of happiness.

CNPQ, CAPES and UFG for promoting research in this country. To everyone who contributed in any way to the completion of this work.

"May I never lose the desire to be big, even though I know the world is small..."

Francisco Cândido Xavier

SUMMARY

The porcine circovirus and associated diseases (PCVAD) syndrome has been described in various regions of the world. Its primary agent, porcine circovirus type 2 (PCV2), is associated with high culling rates on farms and significant economic losses. Several risk factors are related to the manifestation of the clinical symptoms of the syndrome, namely management deficiencies, the presence of co-infections, immunization against the agent and immunostimulation. Among the frequently reported agents associated with PCV2 are porcine parvovirus (PPV) and *Mycoplasma hyopneumoniae*. The aim of this study was to verify the occurrence of PPV and *M. hyopneumoniae,* or co-infection with both, in animals diagnosed with PCVAD in intensive pig production systems in the state of Goiás. Serum and feces samples from 47 animals previously confirmed to be affected by PCVAD were tested for antibodies and PPV DNA, respectively. Nasal secretion samples from 40 animals were analyzed for *Mycoplasma hyopneumoniae* DNA. Of the total number of animals, 20 were euthanized and samples of the spleen, liver, lungs, kidneys, tonsils, intestines and lymph nodes were analyzed in a *pool* for PPV. Seropositivity for PPV was observed in all the sera analyzed, but no genetic material from the same virus was found in the stool samples or in the *pool of* organs analyzed. Of all the nasal secretion samples, six (15.0%) were PCR positive for *Mycoplasma hyopneumoniae*. The results related to the presence of mycoplasma were in line with the clinical findings of the animals analyzed, which presented symptoms of respiratory pathologies and lesions related to the respiratory tract. This was the first report of the association of PCV2 with M. *hyopneumoniae* in pigs identified with PCVAD in the state of Goiás and, to our knowledge, in Brazil.

Keywords: Multifactorial diseases, mycoplasmosis, parvovirosis

1. INTRODUCTION

Brazil occupies a prominent position in world agribusiness. Low production costs and improved zootechnical indices are major factors in maintaining this status.

Brazilian pig farming has been increasing its participation in the global scenario due to the intensification of production systems that give the sector greater profitability and an increase in production efficiency. However, health challenges continue to hinder the optimization of zootechnical results, reducing the competitiveness of the Brazilian market.

The diseases that have the greatest impact on pig farming are those that cause a reduction in the pigs' performance, as they spend more time on the farm before reaching slaughter weight. In addition, the cost of medicines and the depreciation and/or condemnation of carcasses in slaughterhouses must also be taken into account.

Among the main challenges, the porcine circovirus associated diseases (PCVAD) syndrome has been described in several countries (SEGALES et al., 2005). Its primary agent, porcine circovirus type 2 (PCV2), is associated with increased mortality, decreased animal performance and high culling rates (LÓPEZ-SORIA et al., 2005), as well as reproductive failure in pigs (SANCHEZ et al., 2001; LEFEBVRE et al., 2008).

In the majority of clinical cases, it can be proven that PCV2 is necessary, but not exclusive, to cause the circovirus syndrome, and that co-infections (other microorganisms) and other factors (genetics, stress, nutrition and management) are important for the manifestation of the clinical picture (ELLIS et al., 2003; PESCADOR et al., 2003; CIACCI-ZANELLA et al., 2009). In this scenario, the agents that predispose to the occurrence of syndromes associated with swine circovirus should be considered. Among these, the most frequently reported pathogens in Brazil are porcine parvovirus (PPV) and *Mycoplasma hyopneumoniae*.

PPV is endemic in pig populations around the world and is often associated with fetal losses. PPV infection is usually inapparent with the development of immunity and is rarely associated with clinical signs in adult pigs.

Mycoplasma hyopneumoniae is the main causative agent of porcine enzootic pneumonia (PES), a disease characterized by high morbidity and low lethality. Due to its pathogenicity, *M. hyopneumoniae* predisposes its host to secondary pathogens, including PCV2, both of which are involved in the porcine respiratory disease complex (PRDC).

Given the endemicity of PCV2 and *M. hyopneumoniae* in several pig farms in Brazil, the interaction between the agents in animals affected by PCVAD should be analyzed.

Most Brazilian farms test positive for PCV2 in diagnostic tests. Studies have shown an association between PCV2 and PPV, especially in aborted and stillborn fetuses (PESCADOR et al., 2007; ROCHA et al., 2010), and between *M. hyopneumoniae* and PCV2 (CARRIJO, 2012). However, due to the scarcity of data on co-infection between these agents in pigs in Brazil, further studies should be carried out (PESCADOR et al., 2007).

In view of the above, the aim of this study was to identify the presence of PPV and *M. hyopneumoniae* in clinical samples from pigs diagnosed with circovirus in intensive pig production systems in the state of Goiás, in order to provide information on the occurrence and association between these agents.

2. LITERATURE REVIEW

2.1 Porcine circovirus

2.1.1 History

The porcine circovirus (PCV) was first reported by Tischer et al. (1974), using electron microscopy, when they observed a virus morphologically similar to a picornavirus, which caused persistent infection in porcine kidney cell culture (PK-15), without inducing a cytopathic effect. Subsequently, it was shown that this virus had a genome composed of a single, circular, closed DNA strand, which is why it was named porcine circovirus (TISCHER et al., 1982).

Experimental infections with the virus described by Tischer et al. in pigs showed that the agent was eliminated in the animals' feces and nasal secretions, but they showed no clinical signs of disease (TISCHER et al., 1986). In view of these results, studies with the agent became irrelevant.

In 1991, in Canada, a group of animals was observed with progressive weight loss, breathing difficulties, pallor and a lethality rate of approximately 10%. Histopathological examination revealed lesions in the lymphoid system, such as lymphocyte depletion and granulomatous infiltration (SEGALES, 2007).

In 1994, another outbreak of the disease with progressive cachexia, high lethality rates, affecting mainly nursery piglets, and with subacute to chronic evolution was described in pigs, also in Canada (SEGALES, 2007).

In 1998, the genome sequence of the causative agent of the outbreaks described was evaluated and compared to the non-pathogenic virus previously isolated in the PK-15 strain, described by Tischer et al. in 1974. A homology of 68% was observed. As a result, the pathogenic circovirus associated with the reported clinical signs was named porcine circovirus type 2 (PCV2), while the non-pathogenic circovirus became known as porcine circovirus type 1 (PCV1) (MEEHAN et al., 1998; SEGALES, 2007).

Since PCV2 was confirmed as a disease-causing agent, the virus has been identified in several countries, and for some years now it has been considered ubiquitous (CAPRIOLI et al., 2006).

In Brazil, swine circovirus was diagnosed for the first time in 2000. Since then, numerous cases with indications of clinical suspicion of the disease and subsequent laboratory confirmation have been identified, and the circovirus syndrome is currently widespread throughout the country, causing high economic losses for Brazilian pig farming (ZANELLA et al., 2001; PESCADOR et al., 2007).

2.1.2 Etiology

PCV belongs to the *Circoviridae* family, which is subdivided into two genera: *Circovirus* and *Gyrovirus*. Viruses belonging to the *Circoviridae* family have in common icosahedral symmetry and the absence of an envelope. The genome is covalently closed, measuring 15 to 17 nm, and is composed of a single circular strand of DNA, a characteristic unique to this family of viruses, which distinguishes it from other known virus families (TODD et al., 2001).

The *Circoviridae* family is closely related to the *Nanoviridae* family that affects plants, which is why it is thought that the ancestor of PCV1 may have been a plant nanovirus that infected a vertebrate host and recombined with an RNA virus, probably a calicivirus (GIBBS & WEILLER, 1999).

Several small insertions and deletions located throughout the length of the viral DNA genome seem to be responsible for the differences in pathogenicity between PCV1 and PCV2. Both have two main open reading frames (ORFs), called ORF1 and ORF2. ORF1 encodes two replication proteins (rep and rep') and ORF2 encodes the capsid protein - cap (LIU et al., 2006).

In addition to these, ten other ORFs have already been mapped (3, 4, 5, 6, 7, 8, 9, 10, 11 and 12), and some genomic regions of PCV2 have already been identified (WEN, et al., 2012; YANG et al., 2012).

A sequence of 501 nucleotides from ORF2 was analyzed and allowed PCV2 to be divided into two subgroups. The nomenclature adopted in North America divides the genotypes into PCV2a and PCV2b. Studies show that PCV2b is more virulent than PCV2a. In Brazil, both genotypes exist. A third genotype called PCV2c has already been identified and isolated, and has been reported in Denmark (ROWLAND & HESSE, 2009; XU et al., 2012).

2.1.3 . Epidemiology and forms of transmission

PCV2 exclusively affects pigs. Other livestock species (cattle, goats and sheep) have shown no signs of infection by the virus (ELLIS et al., 2003; RODRIGUEZ-ARRIOGA et al., 2003).

The absence of the outer envelope makes PCV2 resistant to alcohol-based disinfectants, chlorhexidine, iodine and phenol. Otherwise, the virus can be inactivated by alkaline disinfectants (sodium hydroxide), oxidizing agents (sodium hypochlorite) and quaternary ammonium compounds (MARTIN et al., 2008). PCV2 has high thermal resistance, maintaining its infectivity when exposed to heat at 75°C for a period of 15 minutes, but is inactivated when subjected to heat at 80°C for more than 15 minutes (O'DEA et al., 2008).

The virus is eliminated from the body in the nasal and oral secretions, urine and feces of infected animals. Sick pigs shed the virus in greater quantities than infected animals that are clinically healthy (HA et al., 2009). Studies in which piglets were monitored from the first week of life until the onset of the disease showed a higher prevalence of PCV2 in nasal secretions than in rectal secretions, supporting the idea that the oro-nasal route is probably the main route of horizontal transmission (GRAU-ROMA et al., 2008).

PCV2 has also been detected in the milk of female pigs, including colostrum, and in the semen of cachaços, in which case there were no changes in the morphology or viability of the spermatozoa

(HA et al., 2009). Despite the presence of the virus in semen, information on the possibility of transmission through this specimen is conflicting. López- Soria et al. (2011) observed that dams inseminated with PCV2-infected semen did not show viremia, nor were antibodies against the virus detected in their bodies, a situation identical to that observed in relation to the fetuses of the dams evaluated. In another study, however, in which gilts from pathogen-free farms were inseminated with semen containing a high concentration of PCV2, there were reproductive failures and PCV2 was isolated from the aborted piglets. It has not been proven whether the concentration of PCV2 contained in semen in natural infections is sufficient to infect sows and piglets (MADSON et al., 2009).

There is evidence that vertical transmission, infection of the embryo or fetus *in utero*, is possible, as identified by the isolation of PCV2 in aborted fetuses, with characteristic lesions in the myocardium (LÓPEZ- SORIA et al., 2008).

Some authors, such as Krakowka et al. (2001), suggest that the development of porcine circovirus-associated syndromes (PCVAD) requires co-infections or co-factors that stimulate the immune system. In support of this line of reasoning, two hypotheses stand out: the first is that co-infections facilitate the expression of PCV2, and the second is that the immunosuppression caused by PCV2 facilitates the expression of secondary pathogens and therefore induces the occurrence of clinical disease.

Epidemiological studies have described the presence of a greater number of other infections or diseases in farms affected by PCV2, such as swine parvovirosis, mycoplasma pneumonia, salmonellosis, Aujeszky's disease, Glasser's disease, *Streptococcus* meningitis, post-weaning colibacillosis and pleuropneumonia (LÓPEZ-SORIA et al., 2008).

2.1.4 Pathogenesis and clinical manifestations

PCV2 has the ability to infect cells of epithelial, endothelial and myeloid origin. *In vitro*, the virus can replicate in some porcine cell lines, and is dependent on cellular proteins expressed during the S phase of the cell cycle. In this way, viral replication *in vivo* is more efficient in tissues with marked mitotic activity. After reaching the lymphatic system, the virus enters the bloodstream and is distributed to the target organs (CASTRO, 2005).

The PCVAD group includes multisystemic swine wasting syndrome (SMDS), porcine dermatitis and nephropathy syndrome (PDNS), reproductive failure, PCV2-associated enteritis, proliferative necrotizing pneumonia (PNP) and congenital tremors (OPRIESSNIG et al., 2007).

MDS is the disease most frequently associated with PCV2. Although there are some non-specific signs, six seem to predominate: cachexia, dyspnea, lymphadenopathy, diarrhea, pallor and jaundice (SEGALES et al., 2004).

Pigs with PDNS show anorexia, depression, prostration, reluctance to move and normal or altered temperature. However, the most obvious feature of the disease is the presence of skin lesions characterized by irregular, red to purple macules and papules, which occasionally coalesce to form large, irregular patches and plaques (CASTRO, 2005).

PNP is a severe form of interstitial pneumonia, characterized by hypertrophy and proliferation of type 2 pneumocytes, and the presence of necrotic cells inside the alveolus (GRAU-ROMA et al., 2008). In enteritis caused by PCV2, the intestinal mucosa is very thickened and the mesenteric lymph nodes are hypertrophied (KIM et al., 2001).

Farms affected by PCV2 have high rates of abortion, mummified fetuses and stillborn piglets. The nucleic acid of PCV2 has been detected in the neural tissue and liver of animals with congenital tremors, which allows the agent to be associated with the disease (SEGALES et al., 2004).

2.1.5 Immunology

The alterations observed in diseases associated with PCV2, such as hypertrophy of the lymph nodes, extensive lymphoid lesions and alterations in the patterns of cytokines released into the blood and lymphoid tissues, which are frequent in clinically affected animals, suggest immune dysfunction and the consequent inability of the animals to produce an adequate immune response (BATISTA, 2009).

The main histological lesion observed consists of lymphocyte depletion to varying degrees, with loss of follicles and the presence of giant multinuclear cells in the lymphoid organs, with multifocal to diffuse distribution. The lesions are related to a decrease in B and T lymphocytes and an increase in monocytes and macrophages in the blood and tissues (ALLAN, 2007).

PCV2 mainly targets antigen-presenting cells: macrophages and dendritic cells (DCs). Although the function of presenting antigens to lymphocytes is maintained, their capacity for antigen recognition is altered (FRANÇA et al., 2005).

A very important characteristic for the manifestation of co-infections is PCV2's ability to interfere with the production of maturation factors by plasmacytoid DCs, thus preventing the activation of T lymphocytes by mature myeloid DCs, resulting in the absence of specific immune responses against other pathogens (MCCULLOUGH et al., 2009).

PCV2 induces the expression of chemotactic factors for macrophages and other inflammatory cells in the affected lymph nodes, thus attracting more mononuclear cells, which will be responsible for the formation of epithelioid macrophages and giant cells, which, in turn, are initiators of the granulomatous inflammatory process also found in animals affected by PCVAD (FRANÇA et al., 2005).

2.1.6 Diagnosis, control and prevention

Due to the widespread presence of PCV2 in the pig population, it is difficult to assess the health status of a farm. For this reason, diagnostic methods which only show the presence of the agent indicate infection, but in no case are they indicative of disease (CASTRO, 2005).

For an individual diagnosis of swine circovirus, the presence of clinical signs, characteristic macro and microscopic lesions in the lymphoid organs (lymphadenopathy and marked lymphocyte depletion with histiocytic infiltration) and the presence of PCV2 DNA or viral antigens must be analyzed together. When diagnosing a herd, individual analysis and epidemiological data from the farm should be taken into account (ALLAN, 2007).

To analyze and correlate the presence of PCV2 in the tissues and histological lesions found, techniques such as immunohistochemistry (IHC) and *in situ* hybridization (ISH) have been used (CHAE, 2004). Although PCV2 is cultivated in some cell lines, it does not produce a cytopathic effect, so the methods for identifying the agent are aimed at detecting the viral genetic content. Due to its high sensitivity and specificity, the polymerase chain reaction (PCR) technique has been adopted to examine specific fragments of PCV2 DNA (ALLAN & ELLIS, 2000; FERNANDES et al., 2006).

In general, farms affected by PCV2 have many management flaws, and the adoption of corrective measures helps to control the causes that lead to the onset of PCVAD. In an attempt to eliminate these inadequate practices, a set of measures was proposed to improve the hygiene of facilities and reduce animal stress. This set of measures has become known as "Madec's 20 points", and includes, among other practices: "all in, all out" management, disinfection, limited contact between animals, no mixing of batches, and isolation or euthanasia of sick animals, among others (MADEC et al., 2000).

As it is a multifactorial syndrome, circovirosis also occurs in farms that follow good production practices, so attention should be paid to controlling concomitant diseases, stimulating the immune system, observing the infection status and the level of antibodies of the female against PCV2 at the time of calving, as well as promoting the constant practice of vaccination (SEGALÉS et al., 2005; ALLAN, 2007; BATISTA, 2009).

Prior to the use of vaccines, which began in 2006, the control of swine circovirus was centered on good production practices. Opriessnig et al. (2007) observed a higher mortality rate in piglets born to sows with viremia and those with low PCV2 antibody levels, meaning that this antibody deficit was directly related to piglet mortality. Piglets that ingest colostrum and have antibodies of maternal origin are less likely to develop PCVAD and have lower lethality rates (LOPÉZ-SÓRIA et al., 2008).

Maternal antibodies, however, only limit viral circulation and excretion and are not totally effective in preventing PCV2 infection. The animal becomes more susceptible to contracting the disease in the time between the decline in antibodies acquired via colostrum and the complete development of active immunity, which occurs around the fifth to eighth week of life (MADEC et al., 2008).

As PCVAD is associated with a strong stimulation of the immune system, Radostitis et al. (2007) hypothesized that vaccines and their adjuvants could aggravate the clinical manifestations of

PCV2, based on the fact that vaccines contain antigens that act as viral or bacterial agents, or even as immunostimulants.

The aforementioned authors also observed that all the adjuvants used at an early stage of infection increased lymphocyte depletion, the duration of viremia and PCV2 levels in the serum (RADOSTITIS et al., 2007).

The appearance of PCV2 vaccines has revolutionized aspects of PCVAD control, showing positive results in terms of reducing lesions and lethality (LOPÉZ-SÓRIA et al., 2008).

Although the vaccination of sows ensures that the piglets receive a high concentration of maternal antibodies, studies by Madson et al.

(2008) indicate that vertical transmission of PCV2 from vaccinated females to their offspring is possible.

2.2 Porcine parvovirus

2.2.1 History

Until the 1960s, reproductive losses in pigs were associated with unknown factors. Environmental, genetic and nutritional factors and toxic agents were considered responsible for low pig production rates (LAWSON, 1961, cited by ROCHA, 2008).

Despite some bacterial agents, and with the advent and development of virus identification techniques, many viral agents have been correlated with reproductive failures. Among them, porcine parvovirus has been identified worldwide with high frequency. This agent was first described in pigs in 1967 and was reported in aborted fetuses in subsequent years. It has been identified as causing disease in pigs in several countries (CARTWRIGHT & HUCK, 1967; RIVERA et al., 1995; ORAVAINEN et al., 2005).

PPV is the agent most commonly linked to embryonic resorptions, abortions, stillbirths, return to oestrus and infertility. The virus is widely distributed in the world's pig population, and farms free of the disease are rare (LIMA, 2010).

2.2.2 Etiology

The name parvovirus was proposed by the International Committee on Viral Taxonomy (ICTV) based on the Latin word *parvus*, which means small, an allusion to the fact that this is one of the smallest viruses identified so far (ANDREWS, 1970; ICTV, 2011).

PPV belongs to the *Parvoviridae* family, in the Parvovirus genus, which has 12 species, all of which are antigenically different from each other. They are small viruses, 18 to 26 nm in diameter, spherical, with an icosahedral capsid and no envelope (MUZYCZKA & BERNS, 2001).

In pigs, only one genus of parvovirus was known, but molecular techniques have made it possible to identify another parvovirus. During a suspected hepatitis E virus infection, a new parvovirus was accidentally identified in pig serum, called porcine parvovirus 2 (PPV2) (HIJIKATA et al., 2001).

In 2007, another virus similar to the parvovirus was identified in pig serum and was named porcine hokovirus (PHoV). The latter and PPV2 have genomes that are phylogenetically distant from the previously known porcine parvovirus, and PHoV and PPV2 have been considered representatives of another genus of the *Parvoviridae* family, which possibly did not originate from PPV (LAU et al., 2008).

The PPV genome consists of a single-stranded DNA molecule, has only four genes and two large open reading frames (ORF). ORF1 encodes three non-structural proteins NS-1, NS-2 and NS-3, which are related to viral replication and the control of gene expression (BERGERON et al., 1993). The NS-1 protein has helicase and nickase activity and is important in viral replication and packaging, and can also induce cell lysis and apoptosis. NS-2 and NS-3 appear to be involved in viral replication (DAEFFLER et al., 2003; SHANGJIN et al., 2009).

ORF2 encodes the three capsid proteins VP-1, VP-2 and VP-3, which are responsible for the structure of the capsid and the adsorption of the virus to the host cell. The substitution of a few amino acids in VP-2 of the viral capsid may be responsible for the difference in pathogenicity between the genotypes (BERGERON et al., 1993; SIMPSON et al., 2002; SHANGJIN et al., 2009).

2.2.3 Epidemiology and forms of transmission

Natural infection by PPV is restricted to pigs. The virus has an affinity for cells with high mitotic activity and depends on cells in the S phase of the cell cycle for replication. This occurs in the nucleus of infected cells during cell multiplication, since the virus has no ability to stimulate or initiate DNA synthesis in resting cells (ROEHE et al., 2007).

Infection by this virus occurs mainly in tissues that have cells with a high capacity for multiplication, such as lymphoid tissues in adults, embryonic cells in pregnant females and precursor cells of the intestinal epithelium in fetuses (MENGELING et al., 1999).

Due to its simple structure, the virus is extremely resistant to environmental conditions, organic solvents, pH changes between 3.0 and 9.0 and heating at a temperature of 60°C for two hours. They can also survive in the environment for up to four months. However, they are sensitive to sodium hypochlorite and 3% formalin (ROEHE et al., 2007).

Due to the viral ability to persist in the environment, facilities containing contaminated secretions and excretions are the main source of infection. Horizontal transmission occurs mainly through oronasal contact, through feces and excrement, from semen and through the vaginal secretions of infected animals. Vertical transmission occurs from the pregnant pig to the litter (WHITTEMORE, 1993).

2.2.4 Pathogenesis and clinical manifestations

Once the virus has entered the body, mainly via the oronasal route, it reaches the bloodstream and replicates in the intestinal crypts, bone marrow and lymphoid tissues, especially the tonsils. Viremia occurs two to four days after infection and persists for two to three days. In breeding stock, PPV causes an infection in the acute phase, clinically inapparent in most cases, and induces a strong immunity. If the infection persists, the virus replicates in intestinal cells and the agent is excreted in the feces of infected animals for long periods, which contributes greatly to environmental contamination (MENGELING et al., 1999; MORAES & COSTA, 2007).

Similarly to PCV2, PPV has a predilection for lymphoid tissues, as a result of which the replication of these agents together can have immunomodulatory consequences, predisposing to secondary infections. PPV also targets the lung and kidney epithelia, hepatocytes and the endothelium. It is important to note that differences in the virulence of viral genotypes are related to tissue tropism (ELLIS et al., 2000).

As PPV has an affinity for multiplying cells, fetuses and fetal envelopes can be infected and become sources of infection (ROEHE et al., 2007). In pigs, the placental barrier is made up of six layers and there is no transposition of antibodies from the mother to the fetus. Otherwise, in the case of transplacental infection, PPV may be carried by blood and lymphatic fluids, by infected lymphocytes and macrophages, or by progressive replication through the tissues that isolate the fetus (MORAES & COSTA, 2007; ROEHE et al., 2007).

The clinical disease occurs mainly in first calving females, which have no immunity to the virus and are at greater risk of infection followed by reproductive problems. In multiparous females who have had previous contact with the agent, the effect of the virus is reduced or null due to the development of active immunity (MORAES & COSTA, 2007).

The spread of the virus is slow, with embryonic or fetal infection occurring within ten to 15 days of infection of the pregnant female. The serious effects of the infection on the body of the infected animal are directly related to the time during pregnancy when the virus is contracted (ROEHE et al., 2007).

When females with low antibody levels acquire the virus during pregnancy, the embryo and fetal envelopes can become infected, predisposing to resorption and abortion. Piglets that ingest colostrum are rarely affected precisely because they acquire protective antibodies against PPV. Passive immunity, however, progressively decreases until the animals reach a lifespan of between four and six months, at which point they become susceptible to infection (MENGELING et al., 2000).

Infected females may show irregular oestrus, fetal mummification, giving birth to fewer young, false pregnancy, decreased weight gain in the final third of the gestational period and smaller abdominal volume during pregnancy (MORAES & COSTA, 2007).

In the early stages of pregnancy, infection usually causes embryonic death and resorption. If most of the embryos die, there may be a return to oestrus, but if most of the embryos remain, the pregnancy can be maintained and a small calf will be born. After ossification, infection of the fetus by PPV also causes death, but resorption is prevented by the fetal skeleton, resulting in mummification (MORAES & COSTA, 2007).

At around 70 days of pregnancy, the fetus becomes immunocompetent and produces its own antibodies, thus surviving the infection. Not all fetuses become infected through the placenta during the viremia manifested by the pregnant woman, as some become infected intrauterinely from adjacent fetuses, a circumstance which highlights a classic feature of the disease: fetal death at different stages of development (ROEHE et al., 2007).

2.2.5 Immunology

The first form of defense used by the immune system against PPV is through physical, chemical and biological barriers. Possibly because it has a simple and compact capsid, capable of withstanding extreme changes in the environment, the virus can easily escape this first barrier (TIZARD, 2002).

The best known form of defense of the immune system against PPV is through the development of specific antibodies to the virus. This active immunity is associated with high and long-lasting antibody titers to PPV, which can be used to monitor herds (JONHSON et al., 1976, cited by SOUZA, 2011).

2.2.6 Diagnosis

The measurement of antibody titers to PPV for diagnostic purposes began to be used in the 1970s, with the standardization of the hemagglutination inhibition (HI) technique (JOO et al., 1976). The distinction between vaccine antibody titers and those derived from the immune response established against PPV in the field can be made by quantifying the level of antibodies, because the humoral stimulation carried out by vaccines generally does not exceed HI titers of 512 (ORAVAINEN et al., 2006).

However, the lack of standardization of serological techniques leads to diagnostic failures, and direct viral detection methods are increasingly being used (ORAVAINEN et al., 2005).

Due to the cytopathic effect (CPE) caused by PPV, viral isolation is a technique used in diagnosis. As a CPE, intranuclear inclusions, pyknotic nuclei, irregular contours, cytoplasmic vacuoles and cell death are observed. However, this technique requires a lot of culture time, which often makes it unfeasible (MENGELING et al., 1999).

Viral DNA can be detected by analyzing tissues from various organs of infected dams, or through fetal tissues from stillbirths, using the PCR technique with primers for the VP2 coding region of PPV. In addition to this technique, nested-PCR was later developed with primers targeting the amplification of the NS1 protein gene, which is more conserved among the different PPV strains (SOARES et al., 1999).

The real-time PCR technique has been described as an efficient form of diagnosis for PPV, as it combines the sensitivity and specificity of conventional PCR with the advantageous possibility of viral quantification (MCKILLEN, 2007).

2.2.7 Control and prevention

There is no specific treatment for PPV. General management measures should be adopted in order to promote good herd health. Vaccination is the main preventive measure adopted, as it aims to stimulate herd immunity, especially in nulliparous cows, avoiding infection of embryos and fetuses (ROEHE et al., 2007).

The vaccines used in Brazil are all inactivated viruses. Vaccination must be carried out on all the farm's breeding stock and varies according to the animal category (replacement piglets, breeding stock in production and male breeding stock) (MORAES & COSTA, 2007).

Colostrum is the only source of antibodies for piglets, due to the placental structure of the female pig, which does not allow the transplacental transmission of antibodies against PPV. Some authors have reported that these passively acquired antibodies can last until the pigs are five months old (MENGELING et al., 1999; FENATI et al., 2009). However, the immunoglobulins responsible for this protection are of the IgG class, and their half-life lasts, on average, around 15 days, which is why Stojonac et al. (2012) believe that, after 30 days of the animal's life, the antibodies found in pig sera come from active immunization against PPV.

2.3 *Mycoplasma hyopneumoniae*

2.3.1 History

The first isolations of *Mycoplasma hyopneumoniae* were made in the 1960s from lung tissue of pigs affected by pneumonia (GOODWIN et al., 1965, cited by VILLARREAL, 2010).

M. hyopneumoniae is the main pathogen of porcine enzootic pneumonia (PES) and, in most clinical events, is associated with secondary bacterial agents and/or viruses, including PCV2. It is estimated that *M. hyopneumoniae* is present in 93% of the world's herds, in which there are low performance indices (CONCEIÇÂO & DELLAGOSTIN, 2006).

2.3.2 Etiology

Mycoplasmas belong to the class *Mollicutes*, a Latin term meaning soft skin. They are the smallest free-living, self-replicating microorganisms known (0.2 µm) and have small genomes (893-920 kpb). Due to the absence of a cell wall, they have a pleomorphic morphology and can take on a spherical, bacillary, helical or filamentous shape (WALKER, 2003).

They have a simple trilaminar membrane made up of proteins, glycoproteins, glycolipids, phospholipids and cholesterol, the latter being responsible for the rigidity and osmotic stability of the membrane. Unlike mycoplasmas that are pathogenic to humans, which are intracellular, *M. hyopneumoniae* is an extracellular microorganism, which is difficult to isolate and cultivate due to its specific nature (ROSS, 1999).

Three groups of *M. hyopneumoniae* isolates were obtained, which were named low, medium and high virulence, based on the host's lung damage score, histopathology, immunofluorescence and serology (VICCA et al., 2003).

M. hyopneumoniae is a very sensitive agent to environmental conditions and is unable to survive for long periods outside its host. In infected lung tissue, it remains infectious for three to seven days in a temperature range between 17 and 25°C. In water, the agent survives for up to 17 days at a temperature range between 2°C and 7°C. On the other hand, its survival time increases in aerosols (SOBESTIANSKY et al., 2007).

2.3.3 Epidemiology and forms of transmission

M. hyopneumoniae is a parasite specific to pigs. Piglets between three and 12 weeks old are more susceptible to infection. The occurrence of the clinical form of the disease is more common in animals in the growing and finishing phases, and in herds lacking immunity, the disease can affect piglets as young as two weeks old, as well as animals in the breeding phase (STARK, 2000).

Transmission between animals occurs horizontally, through direct contact between an infected animal and a susceptible pig, and also indirectly through aerosols from the cough drop of a carrier animal. Vertical intra-uterine transmission and infection through lactation have also been proven, the latter through the consumption of milk contaminated with the agent (STARK, 2000; FANO et al., 2005).

M. hyopneumoniae can also be transmitted through fomites and mechanical vectors. These two transmission hypotheses, however, are of limited importance because they occur less frequently. There is a greater chance of transmission during the winter period, as the weather conditions typical of this time of year favor the agent's maintenance in the environment (BATISTA et al. 2004).

2.3.4 Pathogenesis and clinical manifestations

After penetrating the host organism, mainly via the nasal route, *M. hyopneumoniae* adheres to and colonizes the ciliated epithelium of the trachea, bronchi and bronchioles. This causes agglutination and loss of cilia, with excessive mucus production, thus damaging the mucociliary clearance system and making the respiratory tract more susceptible to opportunistic infections (JACQUES et al., 1992; SORENSEN et al., 1997).

Pathogenic mycoplasmas use a very complex mechanism of pathogenicity, involving adhesion/colonization, cytotoxicity, competition for substrates, evasion and/or modulation of the host's immune response, clastogenic and oncogenic effects (ROSS, 1999).

In pigs, the damage caused by mycoplasma infections is due more to the immune and inflammatory responses elicited by the organism than to the direct toxic effect caused by the cellular components of these microorganisms (RAZIN et al., 1998). *M. hyopneumoniae* interacts with alveolar macrophages and lymphocytes, stimulating them to produce the pro-inflammatory cytokines TNF-α, IL-1 and IL-6, which are responsible for the lung lesions and perivascular and peribronchial lymphoid hyperplasia characteristic of HSP (RODRiGUEZ et al., 2004).

Mycoplasmas are also capable of activating the mitosis of B and T lymphocytes, contributing to the formation of lymphoid hyperplasia, as a result of which the airways become obstructed and atelectatic lesions form in the lungs. These lesions are consolidated and vary in color from purple to gray (SOBESTIANSKY et al., 2007).

The severity of the clinical signs caused by *M. hyopneumoniae* depends on co-infections, as well as environmental and management factors. On farms affected by the disease, disparities in development between piglets of the same age group are common (PIFFER, 1998).

In isolated infections, *M. hyopneumoniae* can cause chronic pneumonia, accompanied by the following characteristic signs: non-productive cough, shaggy hair, increased food intake and reduced growth. When accompanied by other agents, there may also be dyspnea, hyperthermia and prostration (LENEVEU et al., 2005).

2.3.5 Diagnosis

Clinical signs and the presence of lung lesions can be taken as indicative of HSP caused by *M. hyopneumoniae*. Although not pathognomonic, chronic non-productive cough is the most frequently reported sign in affected animals. Lung lesions with a fleshy consistency and a color ranging from gray to purple, usually seen in the cranio-ventral region of the lungs, are frequently observed during necropsy (THACKER, 2004).

The bacteriological culture method is the most accurate for identifying *M. hyopneumoniae*. However, it is rarely used because it is slow, laborious and impractical (VILLARREAL, 2010).

The enzyme-linked immunosorbent assay is used to detect antibodies, but its use is limited since antibodies may only be present in the body of the infected animal for the first six weeks after infection (THACKER et al., 2001).

PCR makes it possible to identify *M. hyopneumoniae* DNA from biological samples of tracheal lavage, nasal secretion and lung fragments. This technique has high sensitivity and specificity, making the identification of the agent faster and more accurate (CALSAMIGLIA et al., 1999; THACKER, 2004; STRAIT et al., 2008).

2.3.6 Control and prevention

PES prevention depends mainly on good management practices. The environment must be suitable, with special attention being paid to air quality, ventilation, temperature and animal density. The separation of animals by age on the farm premises and the "all in, all out" sanitary method are also very important factors (LENEVEU et al., 2005).

Antibiotics are used to treat and prevent *M. hyopneumoniae* infections, but their early or late use at the time of infection can make treatment ineffective. On the other hand, the need to use antiobiotics for prolonged periods of time in certain situations makes the cost of treatment extremely expensive (TIMMERMAN et al., 2006).

Vaccination is a widely used method, although it is not totally effective in preventing infection. Its use promotes a reduction in the number of mycoplasmas in the respiratory tract of pigs, which consequently leads to a reduction in the damage caused by the agent (MEYNS et al., 2007).

In view of the above, and considering the importance of the negative impacts caused by PCVAD in the Brazilian pig herd, this study aimed to elucidate the concomitant occurrence of other agents of importance in pig farming, associated with PCV2.

3. OBJECTIVE

3.1 General Objective

- To evaluate the occurrence of co-infection by porcine parvovirus and/or *M. hyopneumoniae* in pigs from farms affected by swine circovirus syndrome.

3.2 Specific objectives

•   To identify the presence of PPV DNA in samples from pigs with PCV2 in cases of swine circovirus.

•   To identify the presence of antibodies to PPV in pigs affected by swine circovirus.

•   To identify the presence of *Mycoplasma hyopneumoniae* DNA in samples from pigs with PCV2 in cases of swine circovirus.

4. MATERIAL AND METHODS

4.1 Region studied

The samples used in this study came from pigs from six full-cycle farms with a diagnosis of swine circovirus, identified as A, B, C, D, E and F (SALES, 2011; SOARES, 2011), located in the south-central region of the state of Goiás, specifically in the municipalities of Silvânia (A), Paraùna (B), Morrinhos (C), Cristianópolis (D), Inhumas (E) and Senador Canedo (F) (Figure 1). The study was previously approved by the Research Ethics Committee of the Federal University of Goiás (protocol 259/2010).

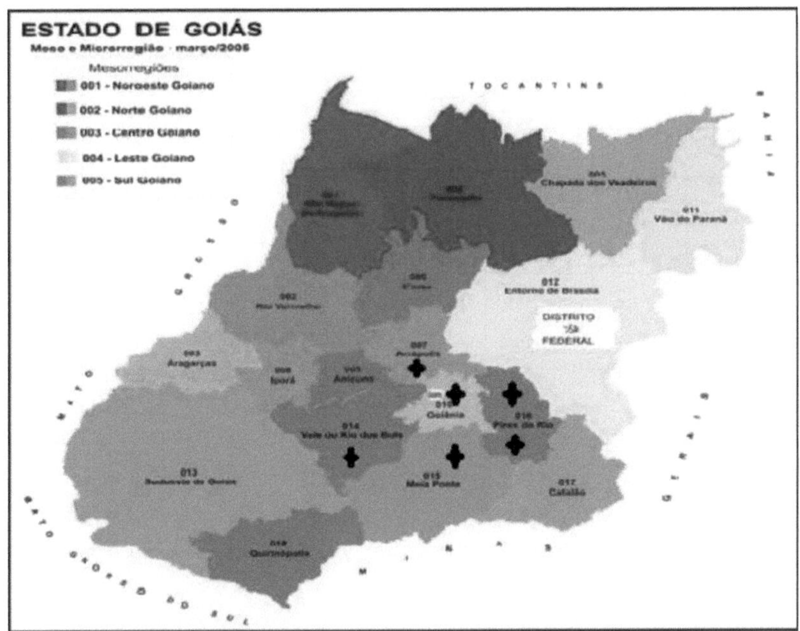

Figure 1: Map of the state of Goiás divided into regions and micro-regions. Black crosses mark the location of the farms. Source: www.seplan.go.gov.br/sepin (SEPLAN/ SEPIN, 2005).

4.2 Sampling

As already mentioned, the samples came from pigs with a clinical suspicion of PCVAD, from farms with high mortality and culling rates, and all the animals, after the appropriate analyses, were diagnosed with the PCVAD syndrome, confirming the previous suspicion (SALES, 2011; SOARES, 2011).

In total, blood, faecal and nasal secretion samples were collected and analyzed from 47 animals, 26 of which came from the nursery phase and the other 21 from the rearing/termination phase (Table 1). Twenty animals (nine from the nursery and 11 from the rearing/termination phase) were necropsied and fragments of the following organs were collected: mediastinal, mesenteric and inguinal lymph nodes, spleen, kidneys, liver, lungs, tonsils and intestines.

TABLE 1 - Number of animals, age in weeks and stage of rearing of animals diagnosed as positive for PCVAD, whose samples were analyzed for identification of PPV and *M. hyopneumoniae*

Farms	Animals	Age (weeks)	Phase
A	1, 2, 3, 4 e 5	6 a 15	2 crèche 3 rearing
B	6, 7, 8 e 9	4 a 8	1 crèche 3 rearing
C	10 e 11	4 a 16	2 rearing
D	12, 13 e 14	4 a 7	3 crèche
E	15, 16 e 17	8 a 9	2 crèche 1 rearing
F	18, 19 e 20	7 a 10	1 crèche 2 rearing
TOTAL 6	20	4 a 16	9 crèche 11 rearing

The methodology described by Sobestiansky et al. (2005) was used to collect the clinical specimens. The animals submitted to necropsy were euthanized using sodium thiopentate (10 mg/Kg) and 10% potassium chloride, applied intravenously, in accordance with Resolution No. 1000 of May 17, 2012 of the Federal Council of Veterinary Medicine (CFMV, 2012).

4.3   Molecular analysis of organ fragments

4.3.1 Extracting DNA from organs

To extract DNA from the tissues, the macerated organs of each animal were first suspended in ultrapure water treated with diethyl pyrocarbonate (DEPC), after which an aliquot of the cell suspension was subjected to DNA extraction using a commercial kit (DNAzol®), according to the manufacturer's instructions (Life Technologies™).

4.3.2 DNA amplification of porcine parvovirus

The protocol developed by Soares et al. (1999) was used to amplify PPV DNA, using a nested-PCR (nPCR) to amplify part of the gene encoding PPV's non-structural NS-1 protein.

Enzymatic amplification was carried out in 50 µl of solution containing 0.5 µM of external oligonucleotides P1 and P6 (Table 2); 2.5 U of Platinum® Taq DNA polymerase; 0.2 mM of each nitrogenous base; 5.0 μl of reaction buffer (500 mM KCl, 15 mM MgCl2, 10 mM Tris-HCl pH 8.0); 5.0 μl of extracted DNA and, as diluent, ultrapure water treated with diethylpyrocarbonate (DEPC). The solution was first heated to 95°C for five minutes in the thermal cycler, then subjected to 35 cycles (95°C for 45 seconds, 55°C for 60 seconds and 72°C for 90 seconds) and 72°C for ten minutes for extension.

In the second stage, a *nested-PCR* (nPCR) was carried out to amplify the internal region of the fragment. This reaction used the internal oligonucleotides P2 and P5 (Table 2), in 25 amplification cycles under the same conditions as described above.

TABLE 2 - Description of the nucleotide sequences of the oligonucleotides used in the nPCR reactions to detect PPV DNA

Reaction	*Primer*	Oligonucleotide sequences	Fragment size (Pb)	Author
PCR	P1	5'-ATACAATTCTATTTCATGGGCCAGC-3'	330	Soares et al., 1999
	P6	5'-TATGTTCTGGTCTTTCCTCGCATC-3'		
nPCR	P2	5'-TTGGTAATGTTGGTTGCTACAATGC-3'	137	Soares et al., 1999
	P5	5'-ACCTGAACGTATGGCTTTGAATTGG-3'		

As a standard positive control for PPV amplification, we used the NADL-2 sample, isolated from the PK-15 strain at the Washington Sugay Swine Diseases Laboratory at the Biological Institute, located in the city of Sao Paulo. Ultrapure water was used as a negative control, to which sterilized DEPC was added.

The products of the nPCR reactions were subjected to electrophoresis in a horizontal vat, on a 1.5% agarose gel with SYBR® Safe dye (Life Technologies™, concentration 10^{-3}), immersed in a 0.5X Tris-borate-EDTA (TBE) cap (0.045 M Tris-Borate, 1.0 mM EDTA), with a voltage appropriate to the size of the gel (1 to 10 V/cm of gel).

The amplified fragments were visualized by transilluminating the gel in ultraviolet light. The sizes of the amplified fragments were compared to a molecular size standard (100 pb DNA Ladder, Life Technologies™), placed on the gel together with the samples analyzed, **and** the necessary controls were carried out for each electrophoretic run.

4.4 Molecular analysis of feces

4.4.1 DNA extraction from feces

A volume of 100 μL of sample was added to microtubes containing 500 μL of lysis solution (Tris-HCl pH 8.0 at 10 mM; NaCl 100 mM; EDTA 2 mM, pH 8.0; 1% sodium duodecyl sulfate and 10 μL of proteinase K at 20 mg/mL). The material was homogenized and incubated at 56°C for two hours. Then 250 µL of phenol and 250 µL of chloroform were added to the mixture, which was homogenized again and then centrifuged at 12,000 x g for ten minutes at 4°C.

The supernatant was then transferred to another 1.5 mL microtube containing 400 µL of propanol. After homogenization, the samples were kept at -20°C for 12 hours. After this period, the samples were centrifuged at 12,000 x g for 25 minutes at a temperature of 4°C.

After discarding the supernatant, the sediment was suspended in 700 µL of 70% ethanol and centrifuged again at 12,000 x g for ten minutes at 4°C. The supernatant was discarded by inversion and the dried sediment was subjected to a dry bath at 56°C for ten minutes. The DNA was suspended in 30 µL of Tris-EDTA (TE) and incubated in a dry bath at 56°C for 15 minutes. The extracted DNA samples were stored at -20°C until they were actually used.

4.4.2 DNA amplification of porcine parvovirus

PPV DNA amplification was carried out using the protocol adapted from McKillen et al. (2007). The *primers* used are described in Table 3. The reactions were carried out in the following stages: heating the sample to a temperature of 94°C for 15 minutes; 35 cycles (94°C for 30 seconds, 57°C for 30 seconds and 72°C for 30 seconds) and a final extension for five minutes at 72°C. The positive control was directed to the beta actin gene, according to the protocol described by Hui et al. (2004).

TABLE 3 - Description of the nucleotide sequence of the oligonucleotides used in the PCR reaction to detect PPV DNA in stool samples

Reaction	Primer	Oligonucleotide sequences	Fragment size (bp)	Author
PCR	F	5'-AAGAGCCTGCTTTGGTGAAA -3'	414	Mckillen et al., 2007
	R	5'-AGAGIIIIGGAGCAAAGGCA -3'		

4.5 Molecular analysis of nasal secretion

4.5.1 DNA extraction from nasal secretion

In microtubes, 500 µL of lysis solution (Tris-HCl pH 8.0 at 10 mM; NaCl 100 mM; EDTA 25 mM, pH 8.0; 1% sodium duodecyl sulfate and 10 µL of proteinase K at 20 mg/mL) were added to 100 µL of sample. The material was homogenized and incubated at 56°C for two hours. Then 250 µL of phenol and 250 µL of chloroform were added to the solution, which was then homogenized and centrifuged at 12,000 x g for ten minutes at 4°C. The supernatant was transferred to another 1.5 mL microtube containing 400 µL of propanol. After homogenization, the samples were kept at -20°C for two hours.

After this period, the samples were centrifuged at 12,000 x g for 25 minutes at 4°C. The sediment was suspended in 900 µL of 70% ethanol, centrifuged at 12,000 x g for ten minutes at 4°C. The supernatant was discarded by inversion and the dried sediment was subjected to a dry bath at 56°C for ten minutes. Finally, the DNA was resuspended in 30 µL of TE solution (10 mM Tris-HCl, 1 mM EDTA, pH 8.0) and incubated in a dry bath at 56°C for 15 minutes. Samples with extracted DNA were stored at -20°C until use.

4.5.2 DNA amplification of *Mycoplasma hyopneumoniae*

Amplification was carried out using the protocol of Artiushin et al. (1993). The *primers* used are described in Table 4. A volume of 2.5 µL of extracted DNA was added to a reaction with a final volume of 25 µL, containing 12.5 µL of DreamTaq™ Green PCR Master Mix (2X), 0.4 µM of each *primer* and DNAse free water q.s.p..

TABLE 4 - Description of the nucleotide sequence of the oligonucleotides used in the PCR reaction to detect *M. hyopneumoniae* DNA from nasal secretion samples

Reaction	*Primer*	Oligonucleotide sequences	Fragment size (bp)	Author
PCR	F	5'- AAGTTCATTCGCGCTAGCCC -3'	483	Artiushin et al., 1993
	R	5'- GCTCCTACTCCATATTGCCC -3'		

The reactions were carried out chronologically in the following order: the sample was initially heated to 94°C for ten minutes, then subjected to 39 cycles (94°C for 30 seconds, 57°C for 30 seconds and 72°C for 60 seconds) and finally subjected to a final extension at 72°C **for** seven minutes.

The nasal secretion samples were tested for the β-actin gene using the PCR method, in order to rule out false negatives, according to the protocol described by Hui et al. (2004).

The amplified fragments were visualized by transilluminating the 1.5% agarose gel in ultraviolet light after staining with *GelRed Nucleic Acid Gel Stain TM* (Biotium, California, USA), according to the manufacturer's instructions. The amplified fragments were compared to a 100 bp marker.

4.6 . Search and titration of antibodies to porcine parvovirus

The identification of antibodies to PPV was carried out using the hemagglutination inhibition (HI) technique, as described by Joo et al. (1976). The antigen used was previously titrated by means of a hemagglutination reaction using guinea pig red blood cells and adjusted to a titre of 4 hemagglutinating units (HU).

Before testing for antibodies, the serum samples were inactivated in a water bath for 30 minutes at a temperature of 56°C and then treated with 25% kaolin solution and guinea pig red blood cells in order to remove non-specific inhibitors. The treated serum was then analyzed against the PPV antigen at 4 HU. The serum was considered positive if it inhibited the agglutination of red blood cells to the PPV antigen. The antibody titer was considered to be the highest dilution of serum that inhibited hemagglutination.

5. RESULTS

After performing PCR on the *pool* of organ fragments and the feces of the animals studied, no sample amplified a PPV fragment (Figure 2).

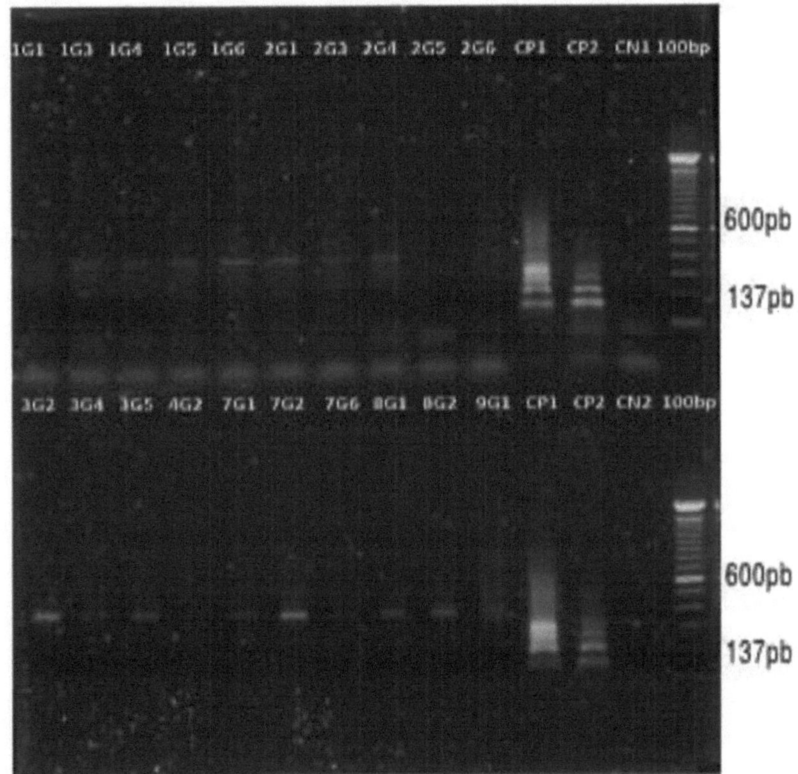

FIGURE 2- Electrophoresis in 1.5% agarose gel. PCR reaction for PPV from the *pool of* tissue fragments obtained from pigs in an intensive production system reacting for PCV2. (PM) Molecular weight 100pb; (CN1; CN2) Negative control; (CP1; CP2) Positive control; (1G1 - 9G1) samples from the 20 animals.

Serum samples from 37 of the 47 animals studied were tested by HI. All (100%) showed the presence of PPV antibodies. The titer of the samples ranged from 1:2 to greater than or equal to 1:256 (Table 5).

TABLE 5 - Results of the PPV antibody titration carried out by

HI technique on serum from 37 animals

Animal	Titration	Results	Animal	Titration	Results
1G1	>1:256	POSITIVE	4G3	1:32	POSITIVE

2G1	1:32	POSITIVE	5G3	>1:256	POSITIVE
3G1	>1:256	POSITIVE	6G3	1:32	POSITIVE
4G1	1:64	POSITIVE	1G4	1:64	POSITIVE
5G1	1:4	POSITIVE	2G4	>1:256	POSITIVE
6G1	1:128	POSITIVE	3G4	1:128	POSITIVE
7G1	>1:256	POSITIVE	2G5	1:8	POSITIVE
8G1	1:4	POSITIVE	1G6	1:4	POSITIVE
9G1	1:2	POSITIVE	2G6	1:2	POSITIVE
2G2	>1:256	POSITIVE	4G6	>1:256	POSITIVE
3G2	1:128	POSITIVE	5G6	1:64	POSITIVE
4G2	>1:256	POSITIVE	6G6	1:64	POSITIVE
5G2	>1:256	POSITIVE	7G6	>1:256	POSITIVE
6G2	>1:256	POSITIVE	8G6	1:16	POSITIVE
7G2	>1:256	POSITIVE	9G6	1:64	POSITIVE
8G2	1:128	POSITIVE	10G6	1:32	POSITIVE
1G3	1:8	POSITIVE	11G6	1:8	POSITIVE
2G3	>1:256	POSITIVE	12G6	1:128	POSITIVE
3G3	1:16	POSITIVE			

Of the 47 nasal secretion samples collected, seven did not present adequate extraction conditions, which is why they were discarded. Of the total of 40 samples tested using the PCR technique, six (15%) (4G1, 7G1, 8G1, 3G4, 1G5 and 3G5) amplified the *M. hyopneumoniae* fragment (Figure 3 and 4) and were considered positive in the diagnostic test.

The six positive samples came from three of the six farms studied (farm A: samples 4G1, 7G1 and 8G1 / farm D: sample 3G4 / farm E: samples 1G5 and 3G5). Of these six samples, three came from animals in the nursery phase (samples 4G1, 1G5 and 3G5) and the other three came from animals in the rearing/termination phase (samples 7G1, 8G1 and 3G4).

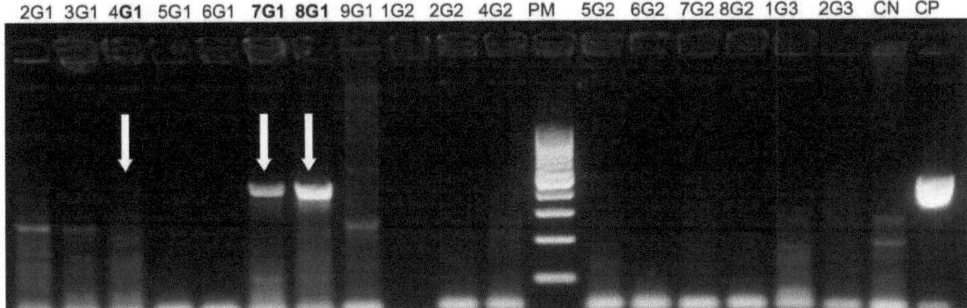

FIGURE 3- Electrophoresis in 1.5% agarose gel. PCR reaction for *M. hyopneumoniae* from nasal secretions. (PM) Molecular weight 100pb; (CP) Positive control; (CN) Negative control; (2G1 - 2G) samples from 17 animals; (4G1, 7G1,8G1) positive samples.

437 pb

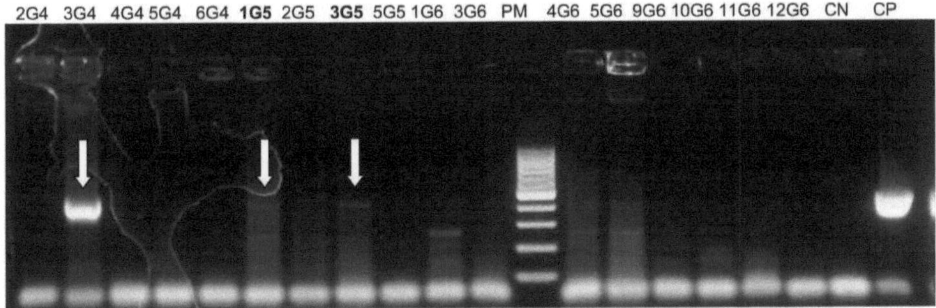

FIGURE 4- Electrophoresis in 1.5% agarose gel. PCR reaction for *M. hyopneumoniae* from nasal secretions. (PM) Molecular weight 100pb; (CP) Positive control; (CN) Negative control; (2G4 - 12 G6) samples from 17 animals; (3G4, 1G5, 3G5) positive samples.

437 pb

29

6. DISCUSSION

The occurrence of PCV2 co-infections with other viral or bacterial agents is well established and has been reported in several studies (CARRASCO et al., 2000; PALLARES et al., 2002; ALLAN et al., 2004; GRAU- ROMA et al., 2011). Among the viral agents most frequently associated with PCV2 for clinical manifestations of PCVAD is PPV. In this study, none of the samples analyzed showed the presence of PPV DNA.

The samples analyzed here were from pigs in the nursery (20 to 63 days old) and rearing (63 to 150 days old) stages. When the history of the herds in which the samples were collected was analyzed (SOARES, 2011), with the exception of the animals from farm D, it was found that all pregnant sows had been vaccinated against PPV before farrowing. According to Mengeling et al. (1999) and Fenati et al. (2009), colostral immunity to parvovirus can last until the animal reaches a life span of between 20 and 24 weeks from the date of birth, a circumstance which may justify the seropositivity of the piglets under study. Undoubtedly, under the conditions of this study, the immunity in question may have contributed to the animals not being infected with PPV.

In the case of farm D, whose sows were not vaccinated, only three of the six sera collected were analyzed, and all of them showed antibodies. In this case, it is inferred that the seropositivity comes from maternal immunity due to previous infection.

The absence of PPV DNA and the presence of anti-PPV antibodies in the animals in this study affected by PCVAD are circumstances that are in line with the results observed by Ostanello et al. (2005), who experimentally inoculated PCV2 and PPV into piglets that ingested colostrum containing antibodies to both viruses. The authors subsequently identified PCV2 genetic material in five of the eight animals inoculated, but did not detect PPV DNA in any of the eight animals, which demonstrates the importance of maternal vaccination as a means of transferring antibodies via colostrum to the offspring. This is particularly important when it comes to the development of infections associated with PCV2 in animals in the nursery and rearing stages, as observed here.

The absence of PPV in the organs of the animals analyzed in this study, however, does not rule out the possibility of the agent being associated with PCV2, given the frequency of parvovirosis in Brazil (BERSANO et al., 1993; BARTHASSON, 2006; STRECK, 2009; LIMA, 2010). Therefore, testing for PPV in events with suspected PCVAD should not be neglected.

In a study carried out in the USA in 2001 and 2002, it was diagnosed that 19.0% of the pigs with SMDS analyzed were co-infected with *M. hyopneumoniae*, which was only preceded in number of cases by porcine reproductive and respiratory syndrome virus (PRRSV) (PALLARES et al., 2002). In Brazil, there are still no records of clinical illness caused by PRRSV, although the occurrence of illness caused by *M. hyopneumoniae is* frequent (SOBESTIANSKY et al., 2007). Although concomitant mycoplasma infection with PCV2 has already been described in the literature in experimental (OPRIESSNIG et al., 2004) and natural (PALLARES et al., 2002) forms, it has not been reported in Brazil to date.

The 15.0% frequency of mycoplasma-positive animals observed in this study is higher than that observed by Sibila et al. (2008) and Nathues et al. (2010), but similar to that described by Moorkamp et al. (2009) and Villareal (2010). According to Marois et al. (2008), tracheobronchial fluids are the most suitable sample for identifying mycoplasma, since *M. hyopneumoniae* attacks the ciliated epithelium of the respiratory tract. However, due to the practicality of the collection procedure, nasal secretions are more often collected using swabs (PIETERS et al., 2009; VILLAREAL, 2010). Therefore, the frequency observed in this study may be underestimated.

In this study, six of the animals analyzed showed the presence of *M. hyopneumoniae* DNA. Of these six, three were from farm A, clinically diagnosed with an outbreak of enzootic pneumonia (data not shown). The other three positive animals came from farms D and E. Of the six farms analyzed, those designated by the letters "A", "D" and "E" did not report the practice of vaccinating for mycoplasma, unlike the other three farms (B, C and F), for which there was a record of vaccination for this agent (SOARES, 2011). Thus, the results obtained here are in line with the immune *status of* the animals. It should be emphasized that, as with PPV, the practice of vaccination is a great ally in animal protection measures, not only against mycoplasma, but also against the occurrence of PCVAD.

Evaluating the clinical and pathological characteristics of the animals used in this study by Sales (2011) and Soares (2011), it was clear that respiratory signs occurred at a high frequency (65%), especially in the animals from farms A, D, E and F. Comparing the results obtained in this study with the data observed in both studies, with the exception of one animal from farm E (sample 1G5), all the other five pigs (samples 4G1, 7G1, 8G1, 3G4 and 3G5) showed respiratory signs, notably coughing (data not shown). According to Opriessnig et al. (2004), coughing is a clinical event present in animals experimentally infected with *M. hyopneumoniae,* or even coinfected with PCV2, but not in animals infected only with PCV2.

Furthermore, among the organs assessed macroscopically, the lung was the one that showed the most alterations in the group of animals analyzed (SALES, 2011; SOARES, 2011). Areas of red hepatization and non-collapsing lungs, lesions described more frequently in animals infected with *M. hyopneumoniae* than in those infected with PCV2 (MORÉS et al., 2007), were observed in 75% of the animals, a finding that suggests the presence of mycoplasma in the farms analyzed (SALES, 2011; SOARES, 2011). Considering the necropsy findings of the euthanized (data not shown) mycoplasma-positive animals identified in this study, they all had the characteristic lung lesions described above.

Lymphadenopathy, another macroscopic finding, absent in pigs infected only with *M. hyopneumoniae,* but evident in animals infected only with PCV2 or with concomitant infection with mycoplasma (OPRIESSNIG et al., 2004), was also observed in the animals evaluated in this study (SALES, 2011; SOARES, 2011).

The clinical and pathological evidence found in the animals analyzed is consistent with the presence of concomitant infection with the agents evaluated, as identified in this study, so that this evidence should be taken as indicative of the presence of mycoplasma in herds with PCVAD, which have not, however, been immunized against this agent.

In this way, and in line with Soares (2011), the results obtained suggest that respiratory diseases, especially those associated with *M. hyopneumoniae,* as identified in this study, may represent the most frequent clinical manifestations in pigs affected by PCVAD in the Goiás State herds studied.

7. CONCLUSIONS

- Under the conditions of this study, within the population analyzed, PPV was not associated with PCV2, and the presence of antibodies in the piglets as a result of vaccination or previous infection of the sows may have played a determining role in the occurrence of this situation;

- This study reinforces the initial assumption that respiratory diseases, especially those associated with *M. hyopneumoniae,* are the most frequently observed pathogens in animals with PCVAD on intensive pig farms in Goiás;

- This was the first study to identify *Mycoplasma hyopneumoniae* in samples from pigs diagnosed with PCVAD in the state of Goiás and, to our knowledge, in Brazil.

8. FINAL CONSIDERATIONS

The data obtained in this study are in line with the results reported in animals affected by PCVAD in several countries and reinforce the epidemiological knowledge about PCV2.

Other agents, which until now had been little studied, have been reported to be associated with PCV2, such as torque teno virus types 1 and 2 (TTV), which have even been diagnosed as co-infecting some of the animals involved in this study (SOARES, 2011).

Other viruses have been described co-infecting animals with the circovirus syndrome and associated diseases, as described by Souza (2011) who made the first report of porcine parvovirus type 2 (PPV2) and porcine hokovirus (PHoV) in pigs with SMDS and by Cibulski (2012) who reported for the first time the presence of porcine bocavirus (PBoV1, PBoV2, PBoV3 and PBoV4) in Brazil associated with PCV2 in animals affected by PCVAD.

However, little data is available on other agents, such as *M. hyopneumoniae*, described in this study, whose presence in Brazilian pig herds is evident. As such, this study represents a scientific contribution to a complex scenario which, with further studies, will have to be definitively resolved.

It is important to carry out a detailed diagnostic investigation of farms where PCVAD occurs, with a view to adopting more efficient intervention strategies. As there are many pathogens involved in the transmission of PCVAD, the mechanism of action of each of them has not yet been properly elucidated, so further, more in-depth studies are necessary to fully understand the syndrome.

One condition that has become clear in this study is the need to vaccinate against preventable diseases such as parvovirus and mycoplasmosis.

9. REFERENCES

1.   ALLAN, G. Advances in PCV2 research - Results of the European Project n° 513928: control of porcine circovirus diseases (PCVDS): Towards improved food quality and safety. In: CONGRESSO BRASILEIRO DE Veterinarios Especialistas em Suinos, 13., 2007, Fiorianópoiis. **Abstracts...** Florianópolis: Brazilian Association of Swine Specialist Veterinarians, p. 125-138, 2007.

2.   ALLAN, G.M.; ELLis, J. Porcine circovirus: A review. **Journal of Veterinary Diagnostic Investigation**, Columbia, v.12, p.3-14, 2000.

3.   ALLAN, G.M.; MCNEiLLY, F.; ELLis, J.; KRAKOWKA, s.; BOTNER, A.; MCCULLOUGH, K.; NAUWYNCK, H.; KENNEDY, s.; MEEHAN, B.; CHARREYRE, C. PMWs: experimental model and co-infections. **Veterinary Microbiology**, Amsterdam, v.98, p.165-168, 2004.

4.   ANDREWs, C. H. Generic names of viruses of vertebrates. **Virology**, New York, v.40, p.1070-1071, 1970.

5.   ARTiUsHiN, s.; sTiPKOViTs, L.; MiNiON, F.C. Development of polymerase chain reaction primers to detect *Mycoplasma hyopneumoniae*. **Molecular and Cellular Probes**, London, v.7, p. 101-105, 1993.

6.   BARTHASSON, D. L. **Molecular identification of porcine circovirus type 2 and hepatitis E virus in pigs from extensive farms in Goiás**. 2006. 90f. Thesis (Doctorate in Animal Science) - Veterinary School, Federal University of Goiás, Goiânia.

7.   BATiSTA, L. A brief review of porcine circovirus. **Solocerdos**, Barcelona: La columna Del investigador, n. 16, p. 3, 2009.

8.   BATiSTA, L.; PiJOAN, C.; RUiZ, A.; UTRERA, V.; DEE, S. Assessment of transmission of *Mycoplasma hyopneumoniae* by personnel. **Journal of Swine Health and Production**, Perry, Iowa, v.12, p.75-77, 2004.

9.   BERGERON, J.; MENEZES, J.; TiJSSEN, P. Genomic organization and mapping of transcription and translation products of the NADL-2 strain of porcine parvovirus. **Virology**, New York, v.197, p. 86 - 98, 1993.

10.   BERSANO, J.G.; SCHOTTEN, M.H.S.; KROEF, S.S.; BASTOS, G.M. Preliminary data on the occurrence of antibodies to porcine parvovirus in the State of Sao Paulo. In: VII Reuniao Anual do Instituto Biològico, **Anais...**, Sao Paulo, v.30, p.17, 1993.

11.   CALSAMIGLIA, M.; PiJOAN, C.; TRIGO, A. Application of a nested polymerase chain reaction assay to detect *Mycoplasma hyopneumoniae* from nasal swabs. **Journal of Veterinary Diagnostic Investigation**, Columbia, v.11, p.246-251, 1999.

12.   CAPRIOLI, A.; MCNEILLY, F.; MCNAIR, I.; LAGAN-TREGASKIS, P.; ELLIS, J.;

KRAKOWKA, S.; MCKILLEN, J.; OSTANELLO, F.; ALLAN, G. PCR detection of porcine circovirus type 2 (PCV2) DNA in blood, tonsillar and faecal swabs from experimentally infected pigs. **Research in Veterinary Science**, London, v. 81, pg. 287-292, 2006.

13.	CARRASCO, L.; SEGALES, J.; BAUTISTA, M.J.; GOMEZ- VILLAMANDOS, J.C.; ROSELL, C.; RUIZ-VILLAMOR, E.; SIERRA, M.A. Instestinal chamydial infection concurrent with postweaning multisystemic wasting syndrome in pigs. **Veterinary Research**, Paris, v.146, n.1, p. 21-23, 2000.

14.	CARRIJO, K.F. **Diagnosis of _Mycoplasma hyopneumoniae_ and porcine circovirus type 2 in lung, kidney and lymphoid tissue and of _Leptospira spp._ in pigs slaughtered under sanitary inspection**. 2012. 155f. Thesis (PhD in Veterinary Hygiene and Technological Processing of Animal Products) - Universidade Federal Fluminense, Niterói, RJ.

15.	CARTWRIGHT, S.F.; HUCK, R.A. Viruses isolated in association with herd infertility, abortions and stillbirths in pigs. **Veterinary Record**, London, v.81, p. 196 - 197, 1967.

16.	CASTRO, A.M.M.G. **Genetic characterization of Brazilian samples of porcine circovirus type 2 (PCV-2)**. 2005. 120f. Thesis (Doctorate in Veterinary Medicine) - Faculty of Veterinary Medicine and Zootechny, University of Sao Paulo, Sao Paulo.

17.	CFMV - Federal Council of Veterinary Medicine. Resolution No. 1000, of May 11, 2012. Provides for procedures and methods of euthanasia in animals, and other measures. **Official Journal of the Union**, Brasilia, May 17, 2012.

18.	CHAE, C. A review of porcine circovirus-2 associated syndromes and diseases. **Veterinary Journal**, London, v.169, n.3, p. 326-336, 2004.

19.	CiACCi-ZANELLA, J.R.; SiMON, N.L.; PiNTO, L.S.; ViANCELLi, A.; FERNANDES, L.T.; HAYASHi, M.; DELLAGOSTiN, O.A.; ESTEVES, P.A. Detection of porcine Circovirus type 2 (PCV2) variants PCV2-1 and PCV2-2 in Brazilian pig population. **Research in Veterinary Science**, London, v. 87, p. 157-160, 2009.

20.	CiBULSKi, S.P. **Viral agents potentially associated with multisystemic wasting syndrome in pigs**. 2012. 160f. Dissertation (Master's Degree in Veterinary Sciences), Federal University of Rio Grande do Sul, Porto Alegre.

21.	CONCEIÇÂO, F.R.; DELLAGOSTIN, O.A. Etiopathogenesis and immunoprophylaxis of swine enzootic peumonia. **Ciência Rural**, Santa Maria, v.36, n.3, p. 1034 - 1042, 2006.

22.	DAEFFLER, L.; HORLEIN, R.; ROMMELAERE, J.; NUESCH, J.P. Modulation of minute virus of mouse cytotoxic activities through site-directed mutagenesis within the NS coding region. **Journal of Virology**, Washington, v.77, p.12466-12478, 2003.

23.	ELLIS, J.A.; BRATANICH, A.; CLARK, E.G.; ALLAN, G.; MEEHAN, B.; HAINES, D.M.; HARDING, J.; WEST, K.H.; KRAKOWKA, S.; KONOBY, C.; HASSARD, L.; MARTIN, K;

MCNEILLY, F. Co-infection by porcine circoviruses and porcine parvovirus in pigs with naturally acquired postweaning multisystemic wasting syndrome. **Journal of Veterinary Diagnostic Investigation**, Columbia, v.12, p.21-27, 2000.

24. ELLIS, J.; SPINATO, M.; YONG, C.; WEST, K.; MCNEILLY, F.; MEEHAN, B.; KENNEDY, S.; CLARK, E.; KRAKOWKA, S.; ALLAN, G. Porcine Circovirus 2-associated disease in Eurasian wild boar. **Journal of Veterinary Diagnostic Investigation**, Columbia, v.15, p.364-368, 2003.

25. FANO, E.; PIJOAN, C.; DEE, S. *Mycoplasma hyopneumoniae* prevalence at weaning as a predictor of the groups' subsequent Mycoplasma status. In: **Proceedings of Allen D. Leman Swine Conference**, Minnesota, USA, p. 109-113, 2005.

26. FENATI, M.; ARMAROLI, E.; CORRAIN, R.; GUBERTI, V. Indirect estimation of porcine parvovirus maternal immunity decay in free-living wild boar (Sus scrofa) piglets by capture-recapture data. **The Veterinary Journal**, London, v. 180, p. 262-264, 2009.

27. FERNANDES, L. T.; CIACCI-ZANELLA, J. R.; SOBESTIANSKY, J.; SCHIOCHET, μ. F.; TROMBETTA, C. Experimental co-infection of porcine circovirus type 2 isolated in Brazil and porcine parvovirus in SPF pigs. **Arquivos Brasileiros de Medicina Veterinària e Zootecnia**, Belo Horizonte, v.58, n.1, p. 1-8, 2006.

28. FRANÇA, T. N.; PEIXOTO, P. V.; BRITO, M. F.; MORÉS, N.; CIACCI- ZANELLA, J. R. Outbreak of circovirosis (multisystemic wasting syndrome in weaned pigs) in the State of Rio de Janeiro. **Pesquisa Veterinària Brasileira**, Seropédica, v.25, n.1, p.39-53, 2005.

29. GIBBS M.; WEILLER G. Evidence that a plant virus switched hosts to infect a vertebrate and then recombined with a vertebrate-infecting virus. **Proceedings of the National Academy of Sciences**, Washington, v.96 p. 8022 - 8027, 1999.

30. GRAU-ROMA, L.; CRISCI, E.; SIBILA, M.; LOPEZ-SORIA, S.; NOFRARIAS, M.; CORTEY, M.; FRAILE, L.; OLIVERA, A.; SEGALES, J. A proposal on porcine circovirus type 2 (PCV2) genotype definition and their relation with postweaning multisystemic wasting syndrome (PMWS) occurrence. **Veterinary Microbiology**, Amsterdam, v.128, p.23-35, 2008.

31. GRAU-ROMA, L.; FRAILE, L.; SEGALES, J. Recent advances in the epidemiology, diagnosis and control of diseases caused by porcine circovirus type 2. **The Veterinary Journal**, London, v.187, p.23-32, 2011.

32. HA, Y.; AHN, K.K.; KIM, B.; CHO, K.-D.; LEE, B.H.; OH, Y.-S.; KIM, S.- H.; CHAE., C. Evidence of shedding of porcine circovirus type 2 in milk from experimentally infected sows. **Research in Veterinary Science**, London, v.86, p. 108-110, 2009.

33. HIJIKATA, M.; ABE, K.; WIN, K.; SHIMIZU, Y.K.; KEICHO, N.; YOSHIKURA, H. Identification of new parvovirus DNA sequence in swine sera from Myanmar. **Japanese Journal of Infectious Diseases**, Tokyo, v.54, p. 244 - 245, 2001.

34.   HUI, R.K.H.; ZENG, F.; CHAN, C.M.N.; YUEN, K.Y.; PEIRIS, J.S.M.; LEUNG, F.C.C. Reverse transcriptase PCR diagnostic assay for the coronavirus associated with severe acute respiratory syndrome. **Journal of Clinical Microbiology**, Washington, v.42, p.1994-1999, 2004.

35.   ICTV. International Committee on Taxonomy of Viruses, 2011. Provides on viral taxonomy. Available at: http://ictvonline.org/virusTaxonomy.asp?version=2011&bhcp=1. Accessed on: 09 Nov 2012.

36.   JACQUES, M.; BLANCHARD, B.; FOIRY, B.; GIRARD, C.; KOBISCH, M. In vitro colonization of porcine trachea by *Mycoplasma hyopneumoniae*. **Annales de Recherches Veterinaires**, Paris, n. 23, p.239-247, 1992.

37.   JOO, H.S.; DONALDSON-WOOD, C.O.R.; JOHNSON R.H. A standardized haemagglutination inhibition test for porcine parvovirus antibody. **Australian Veterinary Journal**, Victoria, v.52, p.422-424, 1976.

38.   KIM, J.; HAN, D.U.; CHOI, C.; CHAE, C. Differentiation of porcine circovirus (PCV)-1 and PCV-2 in boar semen using a multiplex nested polymerase chain reaction. **Journal of Virological Methods**, Amsterdam, v.98, p.25-31, 2001.

39.   KRAKOWKA, S.; ELLIS, J.; MCNEILLY, F.; RIGLER, S.; RIGS, D. M.; ALLAN, G. Activation of the immune system is the pivotal event in production of wasting disease in pigs infected with PCV2. **Veterinary Pathology**, Basel, v.38, n.1, p.31-42, 2001.

40.   LAU, S. K.; WOO, P. C.; TSE, H.; FU, C. T.; AU, W. K.; CHEN, X. C.; TSOI, H. W.; TSANG, T. H.; CHAN, J. S.; TSANG, D.N.G.; LI, K.S.M.; TSE, C.W.S.; NG, T.; TSANG, O.T.Y.; ZHENG, B.; TAM, S.; SHAN, K.; ZHOU, B.; YUEN, K. Identification of novel porcine and bovine parvoviruses closely related to human parvovirus 4. **Journal of General Virology,** London, v.89, p.18401848, 2008.

41.   LEFEBVRE, D.; BARBE, F.; ATANASOVA, K.; NAUWYNCK, H., 2008. Inoculation of porcine foetuses with different genotypes and doses of PCV2. In: INTERNATIONAL PIG VETERINARY SOCIETY CONGRESS, 20, 2008, Durban, South Africa. **Proceedings...** Durban: IPVS, 2008.

42.   LENEVEU, P.; ROBERT, N.; KEÏTA, A.; PAGOT, E.; POMMIER P.; TESSIER, P. Lung lesions in pigs at slaughter: a 2-year epidemiological study in France. **International Journal of Applied Research in Veterinary Medicine**, Apopka, v.3, p.259-265, 2005.

43.   LIMA, E.S. **Serological diagnosis of infectious diseases causing reproductive failure in pigs**. 2010. 113f. Dissertation (Master's Degree in Animal Science). Center for Agricultural Sciences, Santa Catarina State University, Lages.

44.   LIU, J.; CHEN, I.; DU, Q.; CHUA, H.; KWANG, J. The ORF3 protein of porcine circovirus type 2 is involved in viral pathogenesis in vivo. **Journal of Virology**, Washington, v.80, p. 5065-5073, 2006.

45. LÓPEZ-SORIA S.; SEGALES J.; ROSE N.; VINAS M.J.; BLANCHARD P.; MADEC F.; JESTIN A.; CASAL J.; DOMINGO, M. Exploratory study on risk factors for postweaning multisystemic wasting syndrome (PMWS) in Spain. **Preventive Veterinary Medicine**, Amsterdam, v.69, p. 97-107, 2005.

46. LÓPEZ-SORIA, S.; GRAU-ROMA, L.; SEGALES, J. Epidemiologia de la circovirosis porcina. **Suis**, Zaragoza, v.49, p.14-23, 2008.

47. LÓPEZ-SORIA, S.; NOFRAIAS, M.; CALSAMIGLIA, M.; ESPINAL, A.; VALERO, O.; RAMIREZ-MENDOZA, H.; MiNGUEZ, A.; SERRANO, J.M.; CALLÉN, A.; SEGALES, J. Post-weaning multisystem wasting syndrome (PMWS) clinical expression under field conditions is modulated by the pig genetic background. **Veterinary Microbiology**, Amsterdam, v.149, p.352-357, 2011.

48. MADEC, F.; EVEN, E.; MORVAN, P.; HAMON, L.; BLANCHARD, P.; CARIOLET, R.; A MENNA, N.; MORVAN, H.; TRUONG, C.; M AHÉ, D.; ALBINA, E.; JESTIN, A. Post-weaning multisystemic wasting syndrome (PMWS) in pigs in France: clinical observation from follow-up studies on affected farms. **Livestock Production Science**, Amsterdam, v. 63, p. 223-233, 2000.

49. MADEC, F.; ROSE, N.; GRASLAND, B.; CARIOLET, R.; JESTIN, A. Post-weaning multisystemic wasting syndrome and other PCV2-related problems in pigs: a 12-year experience. **Transboundary and Emerging Diseases**, Surrey, v.55, p.273-283, 2008.

50. MADSON, D.M.; PATTERSON, A.R.; RAMAMOORTHY, S.; PAL, N.; MENG, X.J.; OPRIESSNIG,T. Effect of porcine circovirus type 2 (PCV2) vaccination of the dam on PCV2 replication in utero. **Clinical Vaccine Immunology**, Washington, v.16, p.830 - 834, 2008.

51. MADSON, D.; PATTERSON, A.; RAMAMOORTHY, S.; PAL, N.; MENG, X.J.; OPRIESSNIG, T. Reproductive failure experimentally induced in sows via artificial inseminationwith semen spiked with porcine circovirus type 2 (PCV2). **Veterinary Pathology**, Basel, v.46, p.707-716, 2009.

52. MARTIN, H.; POTIER, M.F.; MARIS, P. Virucidal efficacy of nine commercial disinfectants against porcine circovirus type 2. **Veterinary Journal**, London, v.177, p. 388-393, 2008.

53. MAROIS, C.; CARIOLET, R.; MORVAN, H.; KOBISCH, M. Transmission of pathogenic respiratory bacteria to specific pathogen free pigs at slaughter. **Veterinary Microbiology**, Amsterdam, v.129, p.325-332, 2008.

54. MCCULLOUGH, K. C.; RUGGLI, N.; SUMMERFIELD, A. Dendritic cells-At the front-line of pathogen attack. **Veterinary Immunology and Immunopathology**, Amsterdam, v.128, p.7-15, 2009.

55. MCKILLEN, J.; HJERTNER, B.; MILLAR, A.; MCNEILLY, F.; BELAK, S.; ADAIR, B.; ALLAN, G. Molecular beacon real-time PCR detection of swine viruses. **Journal of Virological Methods**, Amsterdam, v.140, p.155-165, 2007.

56. MEEHAN, B.M.; MCNEILLY, F.; TODD, D.; KENNEDY, S.; JEWHURST, V.A.; ELLIS, J.A.; HASSARD, L.E.; CLARK, E.G.; HAINES, D.M.; ALLAN, G.M. Characterization of novel circovirus DNAs associated with wasting syndromes in pigs. **Journal of General Virology**, London, v.79, p. 2171-2179, 1998.

57. MENGELING, W.L.; B.E.; D'ALLAIRE, S.; TAYLOR, D.J. Porcine Parvovirus. **Diseases of Swine**, Ames, 8.ed. Chap.8, p. 119-124, 1999.

58. MENGELING, W.L.; LAGER, K.M.; VORWALD, A.C. The effect of porcine parvovirus and porcine reproductive and respiratory syndrome virus on porcine reproductive performance. **Animal Reproduction Science**, Amsterdam, v.60 - 61, p. 199-210, 2000.

59. MEYNS, T.; MAES, D.; CALUS, D.; RIBBENS, S.; DEWULF, J.; CHIERS, K.; KRUIF, A.; COX, E.; DECOSTERE, A.; HAESEBROUCK, F. Interactions of highly and low virulent *Mycoplasma hyopneumoniae* isolates with the respiratory tract of pigs. **Veterinary Microbiology**, Amsterdam, v.20, p.8795, 2007.

60. MOORKAMP, L.; HEWICKER-TRAUTWEIN, M.; BEILAGE, E.B. Occurrence of *Mycoplasma hyopneumoniae* in coughing piglets (3-6 weeks of age) from 50 herds with a history of endemic respiratory disease. **Transboundary and Emerging Diseases**, v.56, p.54-56, 2009.

61. MORAES M.P.; COSTA, P.R.S. Parvoviridae. In: FLORES, E. (Org.). **Virologia Veterinària**, Santa Maria, p. 275-296, 2007.

62. MORÉS, N.; BARCELLOS, D.; ZANELLA, J.C. Swine circovirus. In: SOBESTIANSKY, J.; BARCELLOS, D. **Diseases of Pigs**. Cânone editorial, 768p, Goiânia, p. 213-226, 2007.

63. MUZYCZKA, N.; BERNS, K.I. Parvoviridae: the viruses and their replication. In: GRIFFIN, D.M.; MARTIN, M.A.; ROIZMAN, B.; STRAUS, S.E. **Fields Virology,** San Francisco, v.2, 4 ed, Lippincott Williams & Wilkins, p. 2327-2359, 2001.

64. NATHUES, H.; STRUTZBERG-MINDER, K.; KREIENBROCK, L.; GROSSE, E.B. Occurrence of *Mycoplasma hyopneumoniae* infections in suckling and nursery pigs in a region of high pig density. **Veterinary Record**, London, v.13, p.194-198, 2010.

65. O'DEA, M.A.; HUGHES, A.P.; DAVIES, L.J.; MUHLING, J.; BUDDLE, R.; WILCOX, G.E. Thermal stability of porcine circovirus type 2 in cell culture. **Journal of Virological Methods**, Amsterdam, v.147, p. 61-66, 2008.

66. OPRIESSNIG, T.; MENG, X. J.; HALBUR, P. G. Porcine circovirus type 2-associated disease: Update on current terminology, clinical manifestations, pathogenesis,diagnosis, and intervention strategies. **Journal of Veterinary Diagnostic Investigation**, Columbia, v.19, p.591-615, 2007.

67. OPRIESSNIG, T.; THACKER, E. L.; YU, S.; FENAUX, M.; MENG, X.J.; HALBUR, P. G. Experimental Reproduction of Postweaning multisystemic Wasting Syndrome in Pigs by Dual

Infection with *Mycoplasma hyopneumoniae* and Porcine Circovirus Type 2. **Veterinary Pathology**, Basel, v. 45, p. 253 - 255, 2004.

68. ORAVAINEN, J.; HEINONEN, M.; TAST, A.; VIROLAINEN, J.V.; PELTONIEMI, O.A.T. High Porcine parvovirus antibodies in sow herds: prevalence and associated factors. **Reproduction in Domestic Animals**, Berlin, v. 40, p. 57-61, 2005.

69. ORAVAINEN, J.; HAKALA, M.; RAUTIAINEN, E.; VEIJALAINEN, P.; HEINONEN, M.; TAST, A.; VIROLAINEN, J.V.; PELTONIEMI, O.A.T. Parvovirus antibodies in vaccinated gilts in field conditions - results with HI and ELISA tests. **Reproduction in Domestic Animals**, Berlin, v. 41, p. 91 - 93, 2006.

70. OSTANELLO, F.; CAPRIOLI, A.; FRANCESCO, A.; BATTILANI, M.; SALA, G.; SARLI, G.; MANDRIOLI, L.; MCNEILLY, F.; ALLAN, G.M.; PROSPERI, S. Experimental infection of 3-week-old conventional colostrum-fed pigs with porcine circovirus type 2 and porcine parvovirus. **Veterinary Microbiology**, Amsterdam, v. 108, p.179-186, 2005.

71. PALLARES, F.J.; HALBUR, P.G.; OPRIESSNIG, T.; SORDEN, S.D.; VILLAR, D.; JANKE, B.H.; YAEGER, M.J.; LARSON, D.J.; SCHWARTZ, K.J.; YOON, K.J.; HOFFMAN, L.J. Porcine circovirus type 2 (PCV2) coinfections in US field cases of postweaning multisystemic wasting syndrome (PMWS). **Journal of Veterinary Investigation**, Columbia, v.14, n.6, p.515-519, 2002.

72. PESCADOR, C.; ROZZA, D. B.; ZLOTOWSKI, P.; BOROWISK, S. M.; BARCELLOS, D. E. S. N.; DRIEMEIER, D. Main histological lesions associated with circovirus in pigs in the growing and finishing stages in herds in Rio Grande do Sul. In: CONGRESSO BRASILEIRO DE VETERINARIOS ESPECIALISTAS EM SUINOS, 11. 2003, Goiânia. **Abstracts...** Goiânia: ABRAVES, p.105-106, 2003.

73. PEsCADOR, C.A.; BANDARRA, P.M.; CAsTRO, L.A.; ANTONiAssi, N.A.B.; RAVAZZOLO, A.P.; sONNE, L.; CRUZ, C.E.F.; DRiEMEiER, D. Coinfection by porcine circovirus type 2 and porcine parvovirus in aborted fetuses and stillborn piglets in southern Brazil. **Pesquisa Veterinària Brasileira**, Rio de Janeiro, v.27, p. 425 - 429, 2007.

74. PiETERs, M.; PiJOAN, C.; FANO, E.; DEE, s. An assessment of the duration of *Mycoplasma hyopneumoniae* infection in an experimentally infected population of pigs. **Veterinary Microbiology**, Amsterdam, v.134, p.261-266, 2009.

75. PiFFER, i. A.; PERDOMO, C. C.; sOBEsTiANsKY, Y. Efeito de fatores ambientais na ocorrência de doenças. in: sOBEsTiANsKY, Y.; WENTZ, i.; SILVEIRA, P. R. S. **Suinocultura Intensiva: Produçâo, Manejo e Saùde do Heranho.** Brasilia: Embrapa-CNPSA, p.257-274, 1998.

76. RADOSTITS, O.M.; GAY, C.C.; HINCHCLIFF, K.W.; CONSTABLE, P.D. Disease associated with viruses and Chlamydia - I. **In Veterinary Medicine** (pg. 1185-1193). Spain: Saunders

Elsevier, 2007.

77. RAZIN, S.; YOGEV, D.; NAOT, Y. Molecular biology and pathogenicity of Mycoplasmas. **Microbiology and Molecular Biology Reviews**, Washington, v.62, p.1094-1156, 1998.

78. RIVERA, E.; SJOLAND, L.; KARLSSON, K.A. A solid phase fluorescent immunoassay for the rapid detection of virus antigens or antibodie in fetuses infected by porcine parvovirus. **Archives of Virology**, Wien, v.88, p. 19-26, 1986.

79. ROCHA, D.L. **Identification of porcine circovirus type 2 and porcine parvovirus in stillborn and mummified porcine fetuses from farms in Brazil**. 2008. 41f. Dissertation (Master's Degree in Veterinary Sciences) - Federal University of Paranà, Curitiba.

80. ROCHA, D.L.; ALBERTON, G.C.; SANTOS, J.L. Identification of porcine circovirus type 2 and porcine parvovirus in porcine stillbirths and mummified fetuses from swine farms in Brazil. **Ciência Animal Brasileira**, Goiânia, v.11, n.3, p. 600 - 606, 2010.

81. RODRIGUEZ-ARRIOGA G.M.; SEGALES, J.; ROSELL, C.; ROVIRA, A.; PUJOLS, J.; PLANA-DURAN, J.; DOMINGO, M. Retrospective study on porcine circovirus type 2 infection in pigs from 1985 to 1997 in Spain. **Journal of Medicine Veterinary**, Berlin, v.50, p.99-101, 2003.

82. RODRIGUEZ, F.; RAMIREZ, G.A.; SARRADELL, J.; ANDRADA, M.; LORENZO, H.; Immunohistochemical labeling of cytokines in lung lesions of pigs naturally infected with *Mycoplasma hyopneumoniae*. **Journal of Comparative Pathology**, Liverpool, v.130, p.306-312, 2004.

83. ROEHE, P.; SOBESTIANSKY, J.; BARCELLOS, D. Parvovirosis. In: SOBESTIANSKY J. & BARCELLOS D.E.S.N. (Org.). **Diseases of Pigs**, 768 p. Goiânia, ed: Canône, p. 286-293, 2007.

84. ROSS, R.F. Mycoplasmal diseases. In: STRAW, B.E. et al. **Diseases of swine**. 8.ed. Ames, Iowa: Iowa State University, p.495-510, 1999.

85. ROWLAND, R.; HESSE, R. PCV-2 nomenclature: How molecular differences translate to the field. In: ANNUAL MEETING OF AMERICAN ASSOCIATION OF SWINE VETERINARIANS, 40., 2009. Iowa. **Proceedings...** [CD-ROOM], Perry: American Associaton of Swine Veterinarians, p.485-486, 2009.

86. SALES, T.P. **Diagnosis of swine circovirus in intensive farms in the state of Goiàs**. 2011.54f. Dissertation (Master's Degree in Animal Science) - Veterinary School, Federal University of Goiás, Goiânia.

87. SANCHEZ, R.E.; NAUWYNCK, H., MCNEILLY, F. et al. Porcine circovirus 2 infection in swine fetuses inoculated at different stages of gestation. **Veterinary Microbiology**, Amsterdam, v.83, p.169-176, 2001.

88. SEGALES, J. (2007). **History and controversy of the disease** (online)   Available   at

http://www.3tres3.com/buscador/noti.php?sec=circovirosis porcina&id=2040&p alabra clave=historia%20y%20controversia%20de%20la%20enfermedad&b s eccion=todo&ajax=2. Accessed on September 12, 2012.

89. SEGALES, J.; ROSELL, C.; DOMINGO, M. Pathological findings associated with naturally acquired porcine circovirus type 2 associated diseases. **Veterinary Microbiology**, Amsterdam, v.98, p.137-149, 2004.

90. SEGALES, J.; ALLAN, G.M.; DOMINGO, M. Porcine circovirus diseases. **Animal Health Research Reviews**, London, v.6 (2), p.119-142, 2005.

91. SEPLAN. **State Secretariat for Management and Planning.** Available at: http://www.seplan.go.gov.br/sepin/. Accessed on: January 22, 2013.

92. SHANGJIN, C.; CORTEY, M.; SEGALES, J. Phylogeny and evolution of the NS1 and VP1/VP2 gene sequences from porcine parvovirus. **Virus Research**, Amsterdam, v.140, p. 209-215, 2009.

93. SIBILA, M.; BERNAL, R.; TORRENTS, D.; RIERA, P.; LLOPART, D.; CALSAMIGLIA, M.; SEGALES, J. Effect of sow vaccination against *Mycoplasma hyopneumoniae* on sow and piglet colonization and seroconversion, and pig lung lesions at slaughter. **Veterinary Microbiology**, v.127, p.165-170, 2008.

94. SIMPSON, A.A.; HEBERT, B.; SULLIVAN, G.M.; PARRISH, C.R.; ZADORI, Z.; TIJSSEN, P.; ROSSMANN, M. The structure of porcine parvovirus: comparison of related viruses. **Journal of Molecular Biology**, London, v. 315, p. 1189 - 1198, 2002.

95. SOARES, R.M.; DURIGON, E.L.; BERSANO, J.G.; RICHTZENHAIN, L.J. Detection of porcine parvovirus DNA by the polymerase chain reaction assay using primers to the highly conserved nonstructural protein gene, NS-1. **Journal of Virological Methods**, Amsterdam, v. 78, p.191-198, 1999.

96. SOARES, P. **Identification of porcine circovirus type 2 and torque teno virus in intensively farmed pigs in the State of Goiás.** 2011.112f. Dissertation (Master's Degree in Animal Science) - Veterinary School, Federal University of Goiás, Goiânia.

97. SOBESTIANSKY, J.; BARCELLOS, D.; MORENO, A. M.; SOBESTIANSKY, A.; POLEZE, E. **Swine: collecting and sending material to laboratories for diagnostic purposes.** Goiânia: Art 3, p. 122, 2005.

98. SOBESTIANSKY, J.; RISTOW, L.E.; MATOS, M.P.C.; BARCELLOS, D. Mycoplasmoses. In: SOBESTIANSKY J. & BARCELLOS D. **Doenças dos Suinos,** 768 p. Goiânia, ed: Canône, p. 159-169, 2007.

99. SORENSEN, V.; AHRENS, P.; BARFOD, K.; FEENSTRA, A.A.; FELD, N.C.; FRIIS, N.F.; BILLE-HANSEN, V.; JENSEN, N.E.; PEDERSEN, M.W. *Mycoplasma hyopneumoniae* infection in

pigs: Duration of the disease and evaluation of four diagnostic assays. **Veterinary Microbiology**, Amsterdam, v. 54, p. 23-34, 1997.

100. SOUZA, C.K. **Diagnosis of parovirus and study of co-infections by swine viruses. 2011.** 102f. Dissertation (Master's Degree in Veterinary Sciences) - Federal University of Rio Grande do Sul, Porto Alegre.

101. STARK, K. Epidemiological investigation of the influence of environmental risk factors on respiratory diseases in swine - A literature review. **Veterinary Journal**, London, v.159, p.37-56, 2000.

102. STOJONAC, N.; GAGRCIN, M.; STEVANCEVIC, O.; STANCIC, I.; POTKONJAK, A. Passive and active immunity against parvovirus infections in piglets. **African Journal of Biotechnology**, Nairobi, v.11, p.7771-7774, 2012.

103. STRAIT, E.L.; MADSEN, M.L.; MINION, F.C.; CHRISTOPHER- HENNINGS, J.; DAMMEN, M.; JONES, K.R.; THACKER, E.L. Real-time PCR assays to address genetic diversity among strains of *Mycoplasma hyopneumoniae*. **Journal of Clinical Microbiology**, Washington, v.46, p.24912498, 2008.

104. STRECK, A. F. **Detection and characterization of swine parvovirus samples**. 2009. 116f. Dissertation (Master's Degree in Veterinary Sciences) - Federal University of Rio Grande do Sul, Porto Alegre.

105. THACKER, E.L. Diagnosis of *Mycoplasma hyopneumoniae*. **Animal Health Research Reviews**, London, v.5, n.2, p.317-320, 2004.

106. THACKER, E.L., THACKER, B.J., JANKE, B.H. Interaction between *Mycoplasma hyopneumoniae* and swine influenza virus. **Journal of Clinical Microbiology**, Washington, v.39, p,2525-2530, 2001.

107. TIMMERMAN, T.; DEWULF, J.; CATRY, B.; FEYEN, B. G.; KRUIF A.; MAES, D. Quantification and evaluation of antimicrobial-drug use in group treatments for fattening pigs in Belgium. **Preventive Veterinary Medicine**, Amsterdam, v.74, p.251-263, 2006.

108. TISCHER, I.; RASCH, R.; TOCHTERMANN, G. Characterization of papovavirus and picornavirus-like particles in permanent pig kidney cell lines. **Zentralblatt fur Bakteriologie**, Stuttgart, Abt.1 Originale A, v.226, p.153-167, 1974.

109. TISCHER, I.; GELDERBLOM, H.; VETTERMANN, W.; KOCH, M. A. A very small porcine virus with a circular singlestranded DNA. **Nature**, London, v.295, p.64-66, 1982.

110. TISCHER, I.; MIELDS, W.; WOLFF, D.; VAGT, M.; GRIEM, W. Studies on Epidemiology and Pathogenicity of Porcine Circovirus. **Archives of Virology**, Wien, v.91, p.271-276, 1986.

111. TIZARD, I.R. **Veterinary immunology - an introduction**. 6ª edition. Ed. Rocca, Sao Paulo,

532 p., 2002.

112. TODD, D.; WESTON, J.H.; SOIKE, D.; SMYTH, J.A. Genome sequence determinations and analyses of novelcircoviruses from goose and pigeon. **Virology**, New York, v.286, n.2, p.354-362, 2001.

113. VICCA, J.; STAKENBORG, T.; MAES, D.; BUTAYE, P.; PEETERS, J.; DE K.A.; HAESEBROUCK, F. Evaluation of virulence of *Mycoplasma hyopneumoniae* field isolates. **Veterinary Microbiology**, Amsterdam, v.97, 177-190, 2003.

114. VILLARREAL, I. **Epidemiology of *M. hyopneumoniae* infections and effect of control measures**. 2010. 22lf. Thesis (Doctor of Veterinary Science) - Faculty of Veterinary Medicine, Ghent University.

115. XU, S.; LI, J.; YUAN, X. WANG, G.; SHI, J.; WU, J.; CONG, X.; SUN, W.; DU, Y.; CHAI, T.; WANG, J. Complete Genome Sequence of Porcine Circovirus 2b Strain Shandong. **Journal of Virology**, Washington, v.86(24):13885, 2012.

116. ZANELLA, C.J.R.; MORÉS, N.; SCHIOCHET, M.F.; TROMBETTA, C. Molecular diagnosis and characterization of porcine circovirus type 2 isolated in Brazil. **Anais da Abraves**, Porto Alegre, RS, p.97-98, 2001.

117. WALKER, R.L. *Mollicutes*. In: HIRSH, D.C., ZEE, Y.C. **Microbiologia veterinària**. Rio de Janeiro: Guanabara Koogan, p.155-162, 2003.

118. WEN, L.; HE, K.; YU, Z.; MAO, A.; NI, Y.; Zhang, X.; GUO, R.; LI, B.; WANG, X.; ZHOU, J.; LV, L. Complete Genome Sequence of a Novel Porcine Circovirus-Like Agent. **Journal of Virology**, Washington, v.86 (1):639, 2012.

119. WHITEMORE, C.; **Science and practice of pig production**. Spain, Ed. Acribia, 1993.

120. YANG, X.; CHEN, F.; CAO, Y.; PANG, D.; OUYANG, H.; REN, L. Complete Genome Sequence of Porcine Circovirus 2b Strain CC1. **Journal of Virology**, Washington, v.86 (17):9536, 2012.

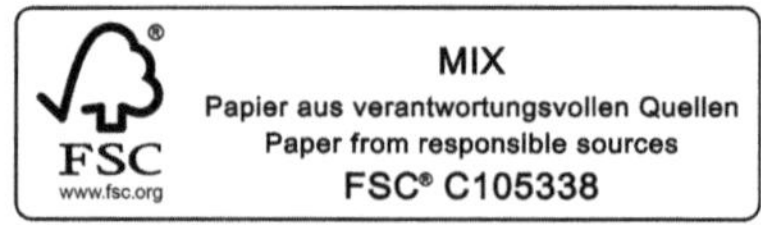

Printed by Books on Demand GmbH, Norderstedt / Germany